Rosacea

Editors

STEVEN R. FELDMAN
LEAH A. CARDWELL
SARAH L. TAYLOR

DERMATOLOGIC CLINICS

www.derm.theclinics.com

Consulting Editor
BRUCE H. THIERS

April 2018 • Volume 36 • Number 2

ELSEVIER

1600 John F. Kennedy Boulevard • Suite 1800 • Philadelphia, Pennsylvania, 19103-2899

http://www.theclinics.com

DERMATOLOGIC CLINICS Volume 36, Number 2
April 2018 ISSN 0733-8635, ISBN-13: 978-0-323-58304-6

Editor: Jessica McCool
Developmental Editor: Sara Watkins

Dermatologic Clinics (ISSN 0733-8635) is published quarterly by Elsevier Inc., 360 Park Avenue South, New York, NY 10010-1710. Months of publication are January, April, July, and October. Business and editorial offices: 1600 John F. Kennedy Blvd., Suite 1800, Philadelphia, PA 19103-2899. Customer service office: 11830 Westline Drive, St. Louis, MO 63146. Periodicals postage paid at New York, NY, and additional mailing offices. Subscription prices are USD 392.00 per year for US individuals, USD 701.00 per year for US institutions, USD 451.00 per year for Canadian individuals, USD 855.00 per year for Canadian institutions, USD 505.00 per year for international individuals, USD 855.00 per year for international institutions, USD 100.00 per year for US students/residents, and USD 240.00 per year for Canadian and international students/residents. International air speed delivery is included in all *Clinics* subscription prices. All prices are subject to change without notice. **POSTMASTER:** Send address changes to *Dermatologic Clinics*, Elsevier Health Sciences Division, Subscription Customer Service, 3251 Riverport Lane, Maryland Heights, MO 63043. **Customer Service: 1-800-654-2452 (U.S. and Canada); 314-447-8871 (outside U.S. and Canada). Fax: 314-447-8029. E-mail: journalscustomerservice-usa@elsevier.com (for print support); journalsonlinesupport-usa@elsevier.com (for online support).**

Reprints. For copies of 100 or more, of articles in this publication, please contact the Commercial Reprints Department, Elsevier Inc., 360 Park Avenue South, New York, New York 10010-1710. Tel.: 212-633-3874; Fax: 212-633-3820; Email: reprints@elsevier.com.

The *Dermatologic Clinics* is covered in *MEDLINE/PubMed (Index Medicus), Current Contents/Clinical Medicine, Excerpta Medica, Chemical Abstracts,* and *ISI/BIOMED.*

Contributors

CONSULTING EDITOR

BRUCE H. THIERS, MD
Professor and Chairman Emeritus, Department
of Dermatology and Dermatologic Surgery,
Medical University of South Carolina,
Charleston, South Carolina, USA

EDITORS

STEVEN R. FELDMAN, MD, PhD
Center for Dermatology Research,
Departments of Dermatology, Pathology, and
Public Health Sciences, Wake Forest School of
Medicine, Winston-Salem, North Carolina, USA

LEAH A. CARDWELL, MD
Department of Dermatology, Center for
Dermatology Research, Wake Forest School of
Medicine, Winston-Salem, North Carolina,
USA

SARAH L. TAYLOR, MD, MPH
Department of Dermatology, Wake Forest
School of Medicine, Winston-Salem, North
Carolina, USA

AUTHORS

CHRISTINE S. AHN, MD
Department of Dermatology, Wake Forest
School of Medicine, Winston-Salem, North
Carolina, USA

HOSSEIN ALINIA, MD
Department of Dermatology, Center for
Dermatology Research, Wake Forest School of
Medicine, Winston-Salem, North Carolina, USA

OLABOLA AWOSIKA, MD, MS
Department of Dermatology, Center for
Dermatology Research, Wake Forest School of
Medicine, Winston-Salem, North Carolina,
USA; Department of Dermatology, The GW
Medical Faculty Associates, Washington, DC,
USA

NAEIM BAHRAMI, PhD
Department of Dermatology, Center for
Dermatology Research, Wake Forest School of
Medicine, Department of Biomedical
Engineering, Virginia Polytechnic Institute and
State University, Wake Forest University,
Winston-Salem, North Carolina, USA

MARC BOURCIER, MD
Hop G. L. Dumont, Dermatology, Dermatology
Clinic, Moncton, New Brunswick, Canada

LEAH A. CARDWELL, MD
Department of Dermatology, Center for
Dermatology Research, Wake Forest School of
Medicine, Winston-Salem, North Carolina,
USA

ABIGAIL CLINE, MD, PhD
Medical College of Georgia, Augusta
University, Augusta University Medical Center,
Augusta, Georgia, USA

STEVEN R. FELDMAN, MD, PhD
Center for Dermatology Research,
Departments of Dermatology, Pathology, and
Public Health Sciences, Wake Forest School of
Medicine, Winston-Salem, North Carolina, USA

ALAN FLEISCHER Jr, MD
Department of Dermatology, Center for
Dermatology Research, Wake Forest School of
Medicine, Winston-Salem, North Carolina,
USA

DENNIS HOPKINSON, MD
Department of Dermatology, Center for
Dermatology Research, Wake Forest School of
Medicine, Winston-Salem, North Carolina, USA

KAREN E. HUANG, MS
Department of Dermatology, Center for
Dermatology Research, Wake Forest School of
Medicine, Winston-Salem, North Carolina,
USA

WILLIAM W. HUANG, MD, MPH, FAAD
Associate Professor, Department of
Dermatology, Wake Forest School of Medicine,
Winston-Salem, North Carolina, USA

SARA M. JAMES, BS
Department of Dermatology, Center for
Dermatology Research, Wake Forest School of
Medicine, Winston-Salem, North Carolina,
USA

LUCY LAN, BA
Department of Dermatology, Center for
Dermatology Research, Wake Forest School of
Medicine, Winston-Salem, North Carolina,
USA

SEAN P. McGREGOR, DO, PharmD
Department of Dermatology, Center for
Dermatology Research, Wake Forest School of
Medicine, Winston-Salem, North Carolina, USA

SONALI NANDA, MS
Department of Dermatology, Center for
Dermatology Research, Wake Forest School of
Medicine, Winston-Salem, North Carolina,
USA

TIMOTHY NYCKOWSKI, BS
Department of Dermatology, Center for
Dermatology Research, Wake Forest School of
Medicine, Winston-Salem, North Carolina,
USA

ELIAS OUSSEDIK, BSc
Department of Dermatology, Center for
Dermatology Research, Wake Forest School of
Medicine, Winston-Salem, North Carolina,
USA

NISHIT PATEL, MD
Department of Dermatology and Cutaneous
Surgery, University of South Florida Morsani
College of Medicine, University of South
Florida, Tampa, Florida, USA

NUPUR U. PATEL, MS
Department of Dermatology, Center for
Dermatology Research, Wake Forest School of
Medicine, Winston-Salem, North Carolina,
USA

IRMA RICHARDSON, MHA
Department of Dermatology, Center for
Dermatology Research, Wake Forest School of
Medicine, Winston-Salem, North Carolina,
USA

MOHAMMED D. SALEEM, MD, MPH
Department of Dermatology, Center
for Dermatology Research, Wake Forest
School of Medicine, Winston-Salem, North
Carolina, USA; University of Florida
Morsani College of Medicine, Gainesville,
Florida, USA

LUCIA SEMINARIO-VIDAL, MD, PhD
Assistant Professor, Department of
Dermatology and Cutaneous Surgery,
University of South Florida Morsani College of
Medicine, University of South Florida, Tampa,
Florida, USA

ALYSON SNYDER, DO
Department of Dermatology, Center for
Dermatology Research, Wake Forest School of
Medicine, Winston-Salem, North Carolina,
USA

JERRY TAN, MD
Schulich School of Medicine and Dentistry, Western University, Windsor Clinical Research Inc, Windsor, Ontario, Canada

SARA MORADI TUCHAYI, MD, MPH
Department of Dermatology, Center for Dermatology Research, Wake Forest School of Medicine, Winston-Salem, North Carolina, USA

JACKSON G. TURBEVILLE, BS
Department of Dermatology, Center for Dermatology Research, Wake Forest School of Medicine, Winston-Salem, North Carolina, USA

LAURA N. UWAKWE, MD
Department of Dermatology, Center for Dermatology Research, Wake Forest School of Medicine, Winston-Salem, North Carolina, USA

NORA VERA, MD
Department of Dermatology and Cutaneous Surgery, University of South Florida Morsani College of Medicine, University of South Florida, Tampa, Florida, USA

JONATHAN K. WILKIN, MD
Department of Dermatology, Center for Dermatology Research, Wake Forest School of Medicine, Winston-Salem, North Carolina, USA

Contents

demographic factors. Subjects were adult patients with a clinical diagnosis of rosacea. Self-assessment severity scores were significantly higher in participants less than 60 years old (mean 3.43 ± 1.07) compared with those greater than or equal to 60 years old (mean 3.09 ± 1.13; $P = .04$). Self-assessment severity scores were significantly higher in men (3.6 ± 1.3) than in women (3.2 ± 1.0; $P = .04$). The authors conclude that rosacea is more severe in men and younger patients.

Rosacea is a common and chronic skin disorder with substantial impact on patients' quality of life. Its varying phenotypic features and facial localization can adversely affect the mental health and socialization of those affected. Although there are no curative interventions, certain therapies have greater effect in improving patient quality of life. This article summarizes the associated psychosocial implications of rosacea. Several skin disease and rosacea-specific quality-of-life measures and their application in clinical care and research studies are also summarized. The recognition and management of the psychosocial impact of rosacea is critical to improving patient outcomes.

Rosacea is a chronic inflammatory cutaneous disorder with an unclear pathogenesis. It has been associated with multiple comorbidities, including cardiovascular diseases, malignancies, depression, migraines, dementia, Parkinson disease, gastrointestinal disorders, and autoimmune conditions. The extent, clinical significance, and implications of these associations remain a topic of discussion. Further evaluation of these comorbidities may offer valuable insight for future screening practices and treatment recommendations.

A variety of triggers are thought to exacerbate rosacea. A validated self-assessment tool and survey was used to study the relationship between rosacea severity and triggers. Subjects were adult patients with a clinical diagnosis of rosacea. Increased severity of disease was significantly associated with consumption of many alcoholic beverages in 1 day and employment at a job requiring extensive sun exposure. The authors' findings may inform physician counseling practices; patients may be provided with practical measures for managing their rosacea, such as limiting alcohol consumption over short periods of time and increasing sun protection, especially in the summer.

Erythematotelangiectatic rosacea is the most prevalent rosacea subtype. Multiple dermatologic conditions may mimic erythematotelangiectatic rosacea. The authors review a comprehensive approach to evaluating subjects with a suspected diagnosis of erythematotelangiectatic rosacea and discuss findings that may warrant further investigation. Differential diagnoses can be narrowed based on the presence of characteristics such as transient erythema, nontransient erythema, and telangiectasias. A thorough history and physical examination are critical in ruling out conditions such as dermatomyositis, lupus erythematosus, atopic dermatitis, and seborrheic dermatitis.

effort to achieve relief. The authors examine the relationship between disease severity and treatment cost across several demographic and socioeconomic strata. Familiarization of evidence-based clinical recommendations and consensus guidelines may equip physicians to educate patients about the most efficacious and cost-effective treatment options to assist patients in making cost-conscious decisions in the management of their rosacea.

Leah A. Cardwell, Timothy Nyckowski, Laura N. Uwakwe, and Steven R. Feldman

Rosacea has significant quality of life impact. The authors review the literature and Internet sources pertaining to rosacea to identify coping mechanisms and resources available to patients with rosacea. MEDLINE and PsycINFO databases were searched to identify pertinent articles. The term "rosacea" was searched in combination with "patient resources," "coping," "dealing with," "blog," "forum," "support," "nonpharmacologic," and "psychological." There are several social and educational coping resources available to patients with rosacea. These may optimize quality of life and psychosocial outcomes in patients with rosacea.

DERMATOLOGIC CLINICS

THE CLINICS ARE AVAILABLE ONLINE!
Access your subscription at:
www.theclinics.com

Preface
Complexities of Rosacea

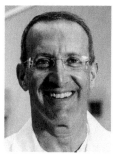 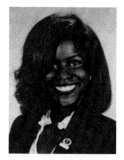 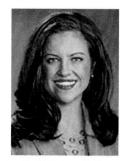

Steven R. Feldman, MD, PhD   Leah A. Cardwell, MD   Sarah L. Taylor, MD, MPH

Editors

Rosacea is a complex dermatologic condition that represents a treatment and management conundrum among many practitioners. Our evolving knowledge of the rosacea disease process has broadened our treatment armamentarium. Though many treatments exist, patients may be recalcitrant to disease or nonadherent to treatment. Frustration with the waxing and waning nature of the condition may prompt patients to neglect their treatment regimens. History of recalcitrant disease, in and of itself, may impact patients' adherence to future regimens. In addition, nonadherence may be misinterpreted as recalcitrance. This may lead to unnecessary escalation of a particular rosacea treatment regimen. To distinguish between the two, optimization of physician-patient rapport is paramount.

Rosacea has tremendous psychosocial impact. Many practitioners underestimate the extent to which rosacea and other dermatologic conditions impact patients. Rosacea affects how patients are perceived, how patients perceive others, and how patients perceive themselves. The condition may be fraught with stigmatization and psychosocial undertones that must also be managed. Careful attention to patient psychosocial status along with rosacea severity status is prudent. The association of rosacea with mental health comorbidities further complicates the situation.

Our goal in this issue of *Dermatologic Clinics* was to review multiple aspects of rosacea, including pathogenesis, clinical presentation, genetic predisposition, epidemiology, treatment, psychosocial burden, comorbidities, triggers, treatment cost, and assessment criteria. We include original research in addition to review articles in an effort to expound upon the rosacea knowledge base.

Steven R. Feldman, MD, PhD
Wake Forest Baptist Medical Center
1 Medical Center Boulevard
Winston-Salem, NC 27157-1071, USA

Leah A. Cardwell, MD
Wake Forest Baptist Medical Center
1 Medical Center Boulevard
Winston-Salem, NC 27157-1071, USA

Sarah L. Taylor, MD, MPH
Wake Forest Baptist Medical Center
1 Medical Center Boulevard
Winston-Salem, NC 27157-1071, USA

E-mail addresses:
sfeldman@wakehealth.edu (S.R. Feldman)
lcardwe@wakehealth.edu (L.A. Cardwell)
saratayl@wakehealth.edu (S.L. Taylor)

Dermatol Clin 36 (2018) xiii
https://doi.org/10.1016/j.det.2017.11.014
0733-8635/18/© 2017 Published by Elsevier Inc.

Rosacea Pathogenesis

Christine S. Ahn, MD*, William W. Huang, MD, MPH

KEYWORDS

- Kallikrein • Cathelicidin • Matrix metalloproteinase • Mast cells • *Demodex*

KEY POINTS

- The pathogenesis of rosacea is not fully understood but involves genetic factors, immune dysregulation, neurovascular dysregulation, and various environmental factors.
- LL-37 (Cathelicidin antimicrobial peptide) and kallikrein 5 are key contributors to immune dysregulation in the skin of patients with rosacea.
- Mast cells are up-regulated and play a role in promoting inflammation.
- Increased activity of transient receptor potential (TRP) cation channels leads to increased levels of vasoregulatory neuropeptides, which mediate flushing in rosacea.
- Skin commensals, such as *Staphylococcus epidermidis* and *Demodex* species as well as bacteria not typically present on the skin, contribute to the pathogenesis of rosacea.

INTRODUCTION

Rosacea is a chronic inflammatory skin disorder with varying prevalence across populations. Affected individuals are typically Fitzpatrick skin type I or II and from northern European or Celtic ancestry. In a Swedish population study, rosacea prevalence was 10%.[1] Rosacea is characterized by the presence of persistent facial erythema with or without edema, telangiectasias, and a tendency for facial flushing and may include inflammatory lesions, eye findings, and skin surface changes over time. Based on clinical characteristics, rosacea is classified into four subtypes, including erythematotelangiectatic rosacea, papulopustular rosacea, ocular rosacea, and phymatous rosacea, although there may be subtype overlap.[2] Histologic findings vary based on the subtype of rosacea, but in inflammatory cases, there are prominent lymphohistiocytic infiltrates around pilosebaceous units and blood vessels.[2] The pathogenesis of rosacea is not fully understood, but genetics, immune factors, neurovascular dysregulation, microorganisms, and environmental factors are thought to play a role (Fig. 1).[3]

GENETIC FACTORS

In a cohort study of twins, a higher correlation of clinical rosacea scores was noted between monozygous twins than between heterozygous twins.[4] In a genome-wide association study, two single-nucleotide polymorphisms were identified in European individuals with rosacea, suggesting that certain genes may predispose to the development of rosacea.[5]

IMMUNE DYSREGULATION

Immune dysregulation is an important component of the pathogenesis of rosacea. Activation of the innate immune system leads to increased production of cytokines and antimicrobial peptides.[3] In patients with rosacea, there are higher baseline levels of cathelicidin and kallikrein 5 (KLK5) in lesional skin.[6] There are a variety of cathelicidins, which have been identified in other mammals, but the only human cathelicidin is human cationic antibacterial protein of 18 kDa (hCAP18).[7] A cathelicidin is an antimicrobial protein, which is stored in the granules of neutrophils and

Disclosure Statement: The authors have nothing to disclose.
Department of Dermatology, Wake Forest School of Medicine, Medical Center Boulevard, Winston-Salem, NC 27157-1071, USA
* Corresponding author. Department of Dermatology, Wake Forest Baptist Health, 4618 Country Club Road, Winston Salem, NC 27104
E-mail address: cahn@wakehealth.edu

Dermatol Clin 36 (2018) 81–86
https://doi.org/10.1016/j.det.2017.11.001

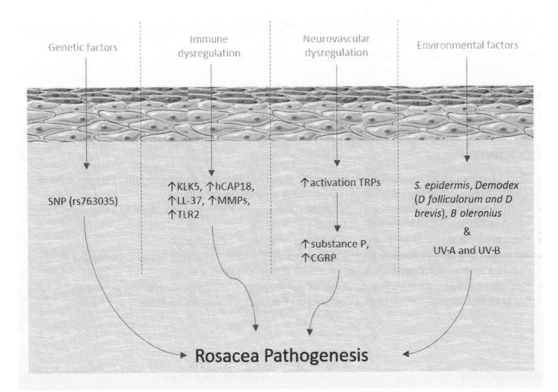

Fig. 1. Schematic of factors contributing to rosacea pathogenesis. An understanding of rosacea pathogenesis is in its infancy; however, hypothesized mediators include genetic factors, immune dysregulation, neurovascular dysregulation, and various environmental factors. hCAP18, human cathelicidin antimicrobial protein; CGRP, calcitonin gene-related peptide; LL-37, cathelicidin antimicrobial peptide, 18kDa; SNP, single-nucleotide polymorphism. (*From* Servier medical art. Available at: http://smart.servier.com/ under a Creative Commons Attribution 3.0 Unported License. Accessed September 8, 2017.)

lamellar bodies of keratinocytes. The inactive protein, hCAP18, is secreted and cleaved into its active peptide form, LL-37, by KLK5 and proteinase 3.[3,8,9] LL-37 has activity against bacteria, fungi, and parasites and is constitutively expressed in neutrophils, mast cells, macrophages, and monocyte granules. In mast cells, LL-37 promotes degranulation and release of inflammatory mediators.[9] In the skin of individuals with rosacea, LL-37 is expressed at higher levels and processed into shorter fragments. The shorter fragments of LL-37 have antimicrobial properties and immune-activating properties; they promote angiogenesis, induce leukocyte chemotaxis, and are involved in the production of proinflammatory cytokines.[10,11] When injected into mice, LL-37 fragments cause erythema, vascular dilatation, flushing, and telangiectasias, symptoms characteristic of rosacea.[6]

Patients with rosacea have higher levels of toll-like receptor 2 (TLR2) and matrix metalloproteinases (MMPs). TLR2, a membrane-bound protein, activates the innate arm of the immune system in response to bacterial, fungal, and viral pathogens. The increased expression of TLR2 on keratinocytes in rosacea-affected skin is the result of

multiple factors, including endoplasmic reticulum stress and the presence of *Demodex*, and leads to higher levels of expression of KLK5 and LL-37. MMPs activate KLK5 via cleavage of the proenzyme. There are increased levels of MMP-2 and MMP-9 in the skin of patients with rosacea, which may lead to increased KLK5 and LL-37 levels.[3,12]

Mast cells likely play a role in rosacea pathogenesis. LL-37, which is secreted by mast cells, influences mast cell activity through induction of chemotaxis, degranulation, and the release of proinflammatory cytokines, including interleukin 6 and MMP-9. In a mouse model study, injection of LL-37 into mast cell knockout mice failed to produce any inflammation. When the mice were reconstituted with mast cells, injection of LL-37 led to inflammation, suggesting that mast cells promote the inflammatory state of rosacea.[3,13,14]

NEUROVASCULAR DYSREGULATION

Transient receptor potential (TRP) cation channels, which are widely expressed on neuronal and non-neuronal cells, such as keratinocytes and endothelial cells, have increased our understanding of the pathophysiology of rosacea. The TRP family of channels consists of two groups, vanilloid (TRPV) and ankyrin (TRPA) receptors. Activation of TRPs leads to the release of mediators of neurogenic inflammation and pain, such as substance P and calcitonin gene-related peptide. These vasoregulatory neuropeptides are critical mediators that induce the sustained flushing that is characteristic of rosacea. The TRPV1 receptor, expressed by sensory nerves and keratinocytes, is expressed in higher levels in patients with rosacea. It is activated by heat, ethanol, inflammatory states, and capsaicin and plays a role in vasoregulation and nociception.[3,15–17] The activity of TRPV1 receptors may explain rosacea patient skin sensitivity and discomfort with exposure to perfumes or herbal extracts, items that may have chemical similarities to capsaicin. TRPV2, TRPV3, and TRPV4 are present on keratinocytes, endothelial cells, immune cells, and neuronal cells. These receptors are present in increased numbers in rosacea-affected skin compared to healthy skin. TRPV2 plays a role in innate immunity, inflammation, nociception, and heat sensing, whereas TRPV3 and TRPV4 are thermosensitive.[16,17] TRPA channels are hypothesized to play a role in the pathogenesis of rosacea by mediating flushing episodes through neurogenic vasodilation. TRPA1 channels, which are thermosensitive, can be activated by cold, formalin, cinnamaldehyde, and mustard oil.[3,8,15,18,19] Rosacea-affected skin had lower heat pain thresholds compared with unaffected skin and rosacea patients had increased burning perception compared with control subjects.[20] This may be due to the increased activity of both TRPV1 and TRPA1 receptors in rosacea.[19]

ROLE OF MICROORGANISMS

Under normal circumstances, the skin has a wide range of commensal organisms, such as *Staphylococcus epidermidis* and *Demodex folliculorum*. Patients with rosacea have notable differences in the composition of the skin flora, including increased burden of skin commensal organisms and presence of bacteria that are not typical members of normal skin flora. It remains unclear whether this dysbiosis of the skin flora is a triggering factor for rosacea or the result of changes in the skin microenvironment in rosacea-affected skin.[3]

S epidermidis is the most common commensal bacteria on the skin. It contributes to the skin host defense by producing antimicrobial peptides, which inhibit the growth of pathogens, such as *S aureus*. In a study assessing the bacterial flora of patients with papulopustular rosacea, there was greater pure growth *S epidermidis* in rosacea pustules compared

with the surrounding skin; the study also noted greater pure growth of *S epidermidis* at the eyelid margins. This suggests that *S epidermidis* may play an integral role in the pathogenesis of pustular and ocular rosacea.[21] *S epidermidis* isolated from rosacea patients was β-hemolytic, this was in contrast to the nonhemolytic *S epidermidis*, which was isolated from control subjects.[22] Hence, *S epidermidis* on rosacea-affected skin may secrete unique virulence factors compared to rosacea-unaffected skin. TLR2 recognizes *S epidermidis* antigens. Interaction between *S epidermidis* and TLR2 leads to downstream activation of KLK5 and promotion of immune dysregulation.[3]

Demodex (*D folliculorum* and *D brevis*) are known commensals of the facial skin. *D folliculorum* tends to favor the hair follicles and *D brevis* is found more often in sebaceous and Meibomian glands. *Demodex* mites have piercing mouthparts and bifid claws that allow them to penetrate cellular membranes and keratin. They perforate cells lining the pilosebaceous follicle and ingest the contents and sebum.[23] In patients with rosacea, there is a higher density of *Demodex* mites on the skin. In one study, *D folliculorum* density was 5.7 times higher in subjects with erythematotelangiectatic rosacea and papulopustular rosacea than in control subjects.[24] In another study, *Demodex* density was higher in subjects with papulopustular rosacea than in control subjects.[25] *Demodex* mites may block the hair follicles and sebaceous glands causing tissue damage. This may lead to increased expression of TLR, recognition of the mites' chitin exoskeletons by immune mediators, and resultant inflammatory reaction. Histologically, this phenomenon is supported by the presence of inflammatory infiltrates around enlarged hair follicles containing *Demodex* mites in rosacea-affected skin.[23] As a survival mechanism, *Demodex* mites may suppress the adaptive immune system by down-regulating T-cell expression.[26,27] *Demodex* mites may perpetuate infestation and hyperproliferation by blocking molecules required for a helper T-cell type 2 response of the adaptive immune response, which leads to release of IL-4, IL-5, IL-6, IL-10, and IL-13.[28] In a study comparing permethrin 5% to metronidazole 0.75% gel, permethrin 5% cream was superior to metronidazole 0.75% gel in reducing *D folliculorum*. The effect of permethrin 5% cream on papules and erythema was comparable to metronidazole 0.75% gel and superior to placebo, but permethrin was not efficacious in the treatment of telangiectasias, rhinophyma, and pustules.[29] These results suggest that *Demodex* are unlikely to be a predominant factor leading to development of rosacea clinical features.[23]

Bacillus oleronius, a gram-negative bacterium, was suggested as a rosacea pathogenic factor after it was cultured from a *D folliculorum* mite in a patient with rosacea.[30] Although its exact role is still unclear, many patients with rosacea have positive serum reactivity to proteins isolated from *B oleronius*. In neutrophils that were exposed to proteins from *Bacillus* species, there were increased levels of migration, increased release of MMP-9 and cathelicidin, and increased production of interleukin 8 and tumor necrosis factor α.[31] Many of these inflammatory mediators and factors are similarly elevated in patients with papulopustular rosacea.[3]

The role of *Helicobacter pylori* and other intestinal bacterial in the pathogenesis of rosacea is unclear. Although some studies report seropositivity of *H pylori* in patients with rosacea, other studies have refuted this.[3,32–34] Regarding the influence of other intestinal bacteria on rosacea, patients with rosacea were thirteen times more likely to have small intestinal bacterial overgrowth (SIBO) compared with control groups. Patients with papulopustular rosacea were twelve times more likely to have SIBO compared with controls. At baseline, 25% of total subjects (n = 22; 20 in rosacea group and 2 in control group) had a positive lactulose hydrogen breath test and glucose breath test and were diagnosed with SIBO; at 3-year follow-up, having completed 10-day treatment with rifaximin, just 5.7% of total subjects (n = 5; 5 in rosacea group and 0 in control group) were positive for lactulose hydrogen breath test or glucose breath test. SIBO diagnosis may be a factor in rosacea development, possibly due to increased circulating proinflammatory cytokines.[3,35]

EXOGENOUS FACTORS

UV radiation is a well-known rosacea trigger. Exposure to UV radiation may cause flushing and worsening of rosacea symptoms. UV-A promotes expression of MMP and causes collagen denaturation whereas UV-B increases production of fibroblast growth factor 2 and vascular endothelial growth factor 2.[36–39] Overexpression of MMP-1 may be involved in the dermal collagen degeneration that is observed in rosacea-affected skin. Compared with healthy controls, rosacea patients have higher levels of reactive oxygen species,[40] which promote production of inflammatory mediators by keratinocytes and fibroblasts. UV radiation induces endoplasmic reticulum stress, which ultimately leads to increased expression of activating transcription 4 and eventual activation of TLR2. An inflammatory cascade is propagated by signaling through TLR2 receptors.[3,41] The tendency of rosacea to affect the central face may be influenced by the preferential exposure of facial convexities to UV radiation.

SUMMARY

The pathogenesis of rosacea is a complex interplay of genetic, immunologic, and neurovascular factors that render individuals susceptible to this chronic inflammatory disease and its many triggers. The treatment of rosacea may be challenging because there seem to be multiple driving factors facilitating disease development. As understanding of the pathophysiology of this complex condition broadens, successful, targeted therapies may be developed.

REFERENCES

1. Berg M, Lidén S. An epidemiological study of rosacea. Acta Derm Venereol 1989;69:419–23. Available at: http://www.ncbi.nlm.nih.gov/pubmed/2572109. Accessed September 2, 2017.

2. Lee WJ, Jung JM, Lee YJ, et al. Histopathological analysis of 226 patients with rosacea according to rosacea subtype and severity. Am J Dermatopathol 2016;38:347–52. Available at: http://www.ncbi.nlm. nih.gov/pubmed/26460622. Accessed September 2, 2017.

3. Two AM, Wu W, Gallo RL, et al. Rosacea. J Am Acad Dermatol 2015;72:749–58. Available at: http://www.ncbi. nlm.nih.gov/pubmed/25890455. Accessed September 2, 2017.

4. Aldrich N, Gerstenblith M, Fu P, et al. Genetic vs Environmental factors that correlate with rosacea. JAMA Dermatol 2015;151:1213. Available at: http:// www.ncbi.nlm.nih.gov/pubmed/26307938. Accessed September 2, 2017.

5. Chang ALS, Raber I, Xu J, et al. Assessment of the genetic basis of rosacea by genome-wide association study. J Invest Dermatol 2015;135:1548–55. Available at: http://www.ncbi.nlm.nih.gov/pubmed/ 25695682. Accessed September 2, 2017.

6. Yamasaki K, Di Nardo A, Bardan A, et al. Increased serine protease activity and cathelicidin promotes skin inflammation in rosacea. Nat Med 2007;13:975–80. Available at: http://www.nature.com/doifinder/10. 1038/nm1616. Accessed September 2, 2017.

7. Larrick JW, Hirata M, Balint RF, et al. Human CAP18: a novel antimicrobial lipopolysaccharide-binding protein. Infect Immun 1995;63:1291–7. Available at: http://www.ncbi.nlm.nih.gov/pubmed/7890387. Accessed September 2, 2017.

8. Chen Y, Moore CD, Zhang JY, et al. TRPV4 moves toward center-fold in rosacea pathogenesis. J Invest Dermatol 2017;137:801–4. Available at: http://www.ncbi. nlm.nih.gov/pubmed/28340683. Accessed September 2, 2017.

9. Niyonsaba F, Kiatsurayanon C, Chieosilapatham P, et al. Friends or Foes? Host defense (antimicrobial) peptides and proteins in human skin diseases. Exp Dermatol 2017;26(11):989–98. Available at: http://www.ncbi.nlm.nih.gov/pubmed/28191680. Accessed September 2, 2017.

10. Koczulla R, von Degenfeld G, Kupatt C, et al. An angiogenic role for the human peptide antibiotic LL-37/hCAP-18. J Clin Invest 2003;111:1665–72. Available at: http://www.ncbi.nlm.nih.gov/pubmed/12782669. Accessed September 2, 2017.

11. Morizane S, Yamasaki K, Mühleisen B, et al. Cathelicidin antimicrobial Peptide LL-37 in psoriasis enables keratinocyte reactivity against TLR9 ligands. J Invest Dermatol 2012;132:135–43. Available at: http://www.ncbi.nlm.nih.gov/pubmed/21850017. Accessed September 2, 2017.

12. Jang YH, Sim JH, Kang HY, et al. Immunohistochemical expression of matrix metalloproteinases in the granulomatous rosacea compared with the nongranulomatous rosacea. J Eur Acad Dermatol Venereol 2011;25:544–8. Available at: http://doi.wiley.com/10.1111/j.1468-3083.2010.03825.x. Accessed September 2, 2017.

13. Margalit A, Kowalczyk MJ, Żaba R, et al. The role of altered cutaneous immune responses in the induction and persistence of rosacea. J Dermatol Sci 2016;82: 3–8. Available at: http://www.ncbi.nlm.nih.gov/pubmed/26747056. Accessed September 2, 2017.

14. Muto Y, Wang Z, Vanderberghe M, et al. Mast cells are key mediators of cathelicidin-initiated skin inflammation in rosacea. J Invest Dermatol 2014; 134:2728–36. Available at: http://linkinghub.elsevier.com/retrieve/pii/S0022202X15365556. Accessed September 2, 2017.

15. Steinhoff M, Schmelz M, Schauber J. Facial erythema of rosacea – aetiology, different pathophysiologies and treatment options. Acta Derm Venereol 2016;96:579–86. Available at: http://www.ncbi.nlm.nih.gov/pubmed/26714888. Accessed September 2, 2017.

16. Pecze L, Szabó K, Széll M, et al. Human keratinocytes are vanilloid resistant. Vosshall LB. PLoS One 2008;3: e3419. Available at: http://www.ncbi.nlm.nih.gov/pubmed/18852901. Accessed September 3, 2017.

17. Sulk M, Seeliger S, Aubert J, et al. Distribution and expression of non-neuronal transient receptor potential (TRPV) ion channels in rosacea. J Invest Dermatol 2012;132:1253–62. Available at: http://www.ncbi.nlm.nih.gov/pubmed/22189789. Accessed September 3, 2017.

18. Pozsgai G, Bodkin JV, Graepel R, et al. Evidence for the pathophysiological relevance of TRPA1 receptors in the cardiovascular system in vivo. Cardiovasc Res 2010;87:760–8. Available at: https://academic.oup.com/cardiovascres/article-lookup/doi/10.1093/cvr/cvq 118. Accessed September 3, 2017.

19. Steinhoff M, Schauber J, Leyden JJ. New insights into rosacea pathophysiology: a review of recent findings. J Am Acad Dermatol 2013;69:S15–26. Available at: http://www.ncbi.nlm.nih.gov/pubmed/24229632. Accessed September 2, 2017.

20. Guzman-Sanchez DA, Ishiuji Y, Patel T, et al. Enhanced skin blood flow and sensitivity to noxious heat stimuli in papulopustular rosacea. J Am Acad Dermatol 2007;57:800–5. Available at: http://linkinghub.elsevier.com/retrieve/pii/S0190962207010274. Accessed September 3, 2017.

21. Whitfeld M, Gunasingam N, Leow LJ, et al. Staphylococcus epidermidis: a possible role in the pustules of rosacea. J Am Acad Dermatol 2011;64:49–52. Available at: http://linkinghub.elsevier.com/retrieve/pii/S0190962209023172. Accessed September 3, 2017.

22. Dahl MV, Ross AJ, Schlievert PM. Temperature regulates bacterial protein production: possible role in rosacea. J Am Acad Dermatol 2004;50:266–72. Available at: http://linkinghub.elsevier.com/retrieve/pii/S0190962203032730. Accessed September 3, 2017.

23. Moran EM, Foley R, Powell FC. Demodex and rosacea revisited. Clin Dermatol 2017;35:195–200. Available at: http://www.ncbi.nlm.nih.gov/pubmed/28274359. Accessed September 2, 2017.

24. Casas C, Paul C, Lahfa M, et al. Quantification of Demodex folliculorum by PCR in rosacea and its relationship to skin innate immune activation. Exp Dermatol 2012;21:906–10. Available at: http://doi.wiley.com/10.1111/exd.12030. Accessed September 3, 2017.

25. Forton F, Seys B. Density of demodex folliculorum in rosacea: a case-control study using standardized skin-surface biopsy. Br J Dermatol 1993;128:650–9. Available at: http://www.ncbi.nlm.nih.gov/pubmed/8338749. Accessed September 4, 2017.

26. Akilov O, Mumcuoglu K. Immune response in demodicosis. J Eur Acad Dermatol Venereol 2004;18: 440–4. Available at: http://www.ncbi.nlm.nih.gov/pubmed/15196158. Accessed September 3, 2017.

27. Akilov OE, Kazanceva SV, Vlasova IA. Particular features of immune response after invasion of different species of human demodex mites. Russ J Immunol 2001;6:399–404. Available at: http://www.ncbi.nlm.nih.gov/pubmed/12687239. Accessed September 3, 2017.

28. Liu Q, Arseculeratne C, Liu Z, et al. Simultaneous deficiency in CD28 and STAT6 results in chronic ectoparasite-induced inflammatory skin disease. Infect Immun 2004;72:3706–15. Available at: http://iai.asm.org/cgi/doi/10.1128/IAI.72.7.3706-3715.2004. Accessed September 3, 2017.

29. Koçak M, Yağli S, Vahapoğlu G, et al. Permethrin 5% cream versus metronidazole 0.75% gel for the

treatment of papulopustular rosacea. A randomized double-blind placebo-controlled study. Dermatology 2002;205:265–70. Available at: http://www.ncbi.nlm. nih.gov/pubmed/12399675. Accessed September 3, 2017.

30. Lacey N, Delaney S, Kavanagh K, et al. Mite-related bacterial antigens stimulate inflammatory cells in rosacea. Br J Dermatol 2007;157:474–81. Available at: http://doi.wiley.com/10.1111/j.1365-2133.2007. 08028.x. Accessed September 3, 2017.

31. O'Reilly N, Bergin D, Reeves EP, et al. Demodex-associated bacterial proteins induce neutrophil activation. Br J Dermatol 2012;166:753–60. Available at: http://www.ncbi.nlm.nih.gov/pubmed/22098186. Accessed September 3, 2017.

32. Rebora A, Drago F, Picciotto A. Helicobacter pylori in patients with rosacea. Am J Gastroenterol 1994;89: 1603–4. Available at: http://www.ncbi.nlm.nih.gov/ pubmed/8079962. Accessed September 3, 2017.

33. Jones MP, Knable AL, White MJ, et al. Helicobacter pylori in rosacea: lack of an association. Arch Dermatol 1998;134:511. Available at: http://www.ncbi.nlm.nih. gov/pubmed/9554311. Accessed September 3, 2017.

34. Sharma VK, Lynn A, Kaminski M, et al. A study of the prevalence of Helicobacter pylori infection and other markers of upper gastrointestinal tract disease in patients with rosacea. Am J Gastroenterol 1998;93: 220–2. Available at: http://www.blackwell-synergy. com/links/doi/10.1111%2Fj.1572-0241.1998.00220.x. Accessed September 3, 2017.

35. Drago F, De Col E, Agnoletti AF, et al. The role of small intestinal bacterial overgrowth in rosacea: a 3-year follow-up. J Am Acad Dermatol 2016;75:e113–5. Available at: http://www.ncbi.nlm.nih.gov/pubmed/ 27543234. Accessed September 2, 2017.

36. Kawaguchi Y, Tanaka H, Okada T, et al. The effects of ultraviolet A and reactive oxygen species on the mRNA expression of 72-kDa type IV collagenase and its tissue inhibitor in cultured human dermal fibroblasts. Arch Dermatol Res 1996;288:39–44. Available at: http://www.ncbi.nlm.nih.gov/pubmed/ 8750933. Accessed September 3, 2017.

37. Naru E, Suzuki T, Moriyama M, et al. Functional changes induced by chronic UVA irradiation to cultured human dermal fibroblasts. Br J Dermatol 2005;153(Suppl 2):6–12. Available at: http://doi.wiley. com/10.1111/j.1365-2133.2005.06964.x. Accessed September 3, 2017.

38. Brauchle M, Funk JO, Kind P, et al. Ultraviolet B and H2O2 are potent inducers of vascular endothelial growth factor expression in cultured keratinocytes. J Biol Chem 1996;271:21793–7. Available at: http:// www.ncbi.nlm.nih.gov/pubmed/8702976. Accessed September 3, 2017.

39. Bielenberg DR, Bucana CD, Sanchez R, et al. Molecular regulation of UVB-induced cutaneous angiogenesis. J Invest Dermatol 1998;111:864–72. Available at: http://www.ncbi.nlm.nih.gov/pubmed/ 9804351. Accessed September 3, 2017.

40. Bakar O, Demirçay Z, Yuksel M, et al. The effect of azithromycin on reactive oxygen species in rosacea. Clin Exp Dermatol 2007;32:197–200. Available at: http://doi.wiley.com/10.1111/j.1365-2230. 2006.02322.x. Accessed September 3, 2017.

41. Woo Y, Lim J, Cho D, et al. Rosacea: molecular mechanisms and management of a chronic cutaneous inflammatory condition. Int J Mol Sci 2016;17: 1562. Available at: http://www.ncbi.nlm.nih.gov/ pubmed/27649161. Accessed September 2, 2017.

Genetic Predisposition to Rosacea

Olabola Awosika, MD, MS[a],*, Elias Oussedik, BSc[b]

KEYWORDS

- Human leukocyte antigen • Single-nucleotide polymorphism • HLA-DRA

KEY POINTS

- The genetics of rosacea are poorly understood; however, gene variants, susceptibility, and associations with other autoimmune diseases provide insight into the genetic predisposition to rosacea.
- Rosacea may have evolved as a genetic mutation during low UV levels to allow vitamin D–independent *CAMP* activation and, thus, provide host defense against microbial infections.
- An overlap of certain genes in the genetic profiles of rosacea subtypes suggests a developmental march from an early inflammatory stage to a hyperglandular-phymatous stage.
- Rosacea is associated with the single-nucleotide polymorphism, rs763035, and the following HLA alleles: *HLA-DRB1*03:01*, *HLA-DQB1*02:01*, and *HLA-DQA1*05:01*.
- Rosacea shares genetic risk loci with autoimmune diseases, including type I diabetes, sarcoidosis, ulcerative colitis, celiac disease, and multiple sclerosis.

INTRODUCTION

Rosacea is a common, chronic inflammatory skin disease characterized by facial flushing and erythema, papules, pustules, and/or telangiectasias. Secondary features of rosacea may include burning and stinging, scaling dermatitis, and edema of the face.[1] This skin disorder is easily identifiable in fair-skinned individuals and may progress to ocular involvement and rhinophyma in severe cases. Although clinical patterns of the disease often overlap, the National Rosacea Society Expert Committee recognizes the following 4 major subtypes of rosacea: erythematotelangiectatic rosacea (ETR), inflammatory papulopustular rosacea (PPR), phymatous rosacea (PhR), and ocular rosacea.[2] This variable clinical presentation of rosacea may be explained by the multifactorial basis of its pathophysiology. Specifically, the etiopathogenesis involves complex interactions within the innate immune system mediated by toll-like receptor 2 (TLR-2) and neurovascular dysregulation mediated by transient receptor potential channel vanilloid receptor 1 (TRPV1).[3] Identified triggers for this pathogenesis include physical (ultraviolet light, temperature), biological (spicy food, microbiota), and endogenous (stress, genetic) stimuli.[4]

Evidence of a family history of the disease in up to one-third of patients with rosacea suggests a strong familial inheritance of the disorder.[1] The higher incidence of rosacea in Celtic and Northern European descendants suggests that there may be a genetic predilection to this disorder.[2] However, the particular role of genetics in the development and persistence of rosacea remains poorly understood. Recent advances in research into gene loci and expression, genetic susceptibility in twin studies, and associations with other autoimmune diseases have provided

Disclosure Statement: The authors have nothing to disclose.
[a] Department of Dermatology, The George Washington Medical Faculty Associates, 2150 Pennsylvania Avenue Northwest, 2B-427, Washington, DC 20037, USA; [b] Department of Dermatology, Center for Dermatology Research, Wake Forest School of Medicine, Medical Center Boulevard, Winston-Salem, NC 27157-1071, USA
* Corresponding author.
E-mail address: olabolaa@gmail.com

Dermatol Clin 36 (2018) 87–92
https://doi.org/10.1016/j.det.2017.11.002

further insight into the genetic predisposition to rosacea.

Genetic Origin

The pathophysiology of rosacea and its predominance among certain populations may be explained by the genetic origin of the disease. One of the most compelling arguments for the genetic predisposition to rosacea is its high incidence in persons of Northern European descent, particularly the Celtic population. It is hypothesized that rosacea developed as a mutation in Celts to adapt protection against life-threatening bacterial infections, such as lupus vulgaris (also known as tuberculosis luposa) during UV-deficient periods.[5] Endoplasmic reticulum (ER) stress and sphigosine-1-phosphate (S1P) signaling in rosacea may have compensated for reduced vitamin D–dependent cathelicidin antimicrobial peptide (CAMP) expression during UV-deficient Nordic winters. Under adequate UVB exposure, UVB leads to 2 actions: (1) activation of the *CAMP* promoter via a vitamin D receptor and (2) induction of ER stress causing conversion of ceramide into S1P and, subsequent, promotion of C/EBPα gene expression of CAMP. This production of CAMP is important, as it provides cutaneous defense against bacterial pathogens, such as methicillin-resistant *Staphylococcus aureus* and *Mycobacterium tuberculosis*, as well as viral and fungal infections.[5–7] Rosacea may have evolved in Northern Europeans under exposure to environmental conditions with insufficient vitamin D–dependent *CAMP* activation. In the absence of UVB, upregulation of CAMP occurs via enhanced ER stress signaling causing intrinsic activation of the alternative C/EBP-α–regulated *CAMP* promoter (transcription factor for CAMP). Multiple rosacea pathologies can be explained by ER stress-driven transcriptional regulations, such as production of S1P and LL37. For instance, the sensation of heat and sebaceous gland dysfunction in rosacea are mediated by S1P sensitization of TRPV1. The development of telangiectasias, UV sensitivity, and inflammation over sebaceous gland–rich areas of the face may result from LL37–mediated angiogenesis and inflammation. Despite this evidence for the linkage of ER stress-driven CAMP production to the etiopathogenesis of rosacea, the genetic defect underlying increased ER stress signaling remains unknown.[5]

Gene Expression and Transcription Studies

The association between gene expression and the manifestation of rosacea has been explored by several population and genetic analysis studies.

Data from epidemiologic studies comparing the prevalence, skin phenotype, and geographic distribution of rosacea suggest a genetic component to rosacea.[8–10] Transcriptome profile analysis has confirmed the existence of selective and overlapping gene profiles for subtypes of rosacea.[10] Consistent with rosacea pathogenesis, genes of the innate immune response are actively expressed in skin lesions of ETR, PPR, and PhR. However, the expression of genes of the adaptive immune response are most prominent in the PPR and PhR subtypes. Gene studies and histologic data do not reveal a significant role for known microbial agents in early phases of rosacea.[10] Rather, the overlap of certain genes in the genetic profiles of rosacea subtypes suggests that a developmental march from an early inflammatory stage to a hyperglandular-phymatous stage occurs in some patients.[3,10]

The genetic profile of rosacea subtypes has also been compared with disorders with overlapping clinical features. In a case-control observational study, gene expression varied greatly between the ETR subtype and telangiectatic photoaging (TP). Despite the shared features of facial erythema and telangiectasia in both entities, 10 genes of selected mast cell-activating neuropeptides, immune modulators, and extracellular matrix components were overexpressed in ETR compared with TP. Fifteen genes were overexpressed in ETR compared with healthy controls (**Table 1**). Identified genes of significance encoded for substance P, matrix metalloproteinases, tumor necrosis factor alpha, and chemoattractants for mast cells (*TAC1*, *MMP9*, *TNFA*, and *CXCL12*, respectively). The demonstrated increased expression of *CXCL12* and its receptor CXCR4 in ETR compared with TP and healthy skin support the important role of mast cell migration and degranulation in rosacea. Substance P is of particular interest, given its known role of vasodilation and increased vascular permeability through action on vascular smooth muscle to release nitric oxide. The greater expression of substance P in ETR may explain the greater frequency of transient and nontransient erythema in ETR compared with TP. The overexpression of MMP9 and genes for type I collagen and type III collagen in ETR, in comparison to both TP and healthy controls, provides further support for the developmental march hypothesis as ECM remodeling directly affects vascular cell biology (as seen in ETR) and MMP gene upregulation is well documented in PPR and PhR.[3,11]

Considering specific gene loci of interest, population studies have identified gene variants associated with rosacea that may provide further insight

Table 1
Genes overexpressed in rosacea (erythematotelangiectatic rosacea) compared with normal skin

Gene	Gene Product
Neuropeptides	
CALCA	Calcitonin-related peptide α
CALCB	Calcitonin-related polypeptide β
TAC1	Tachykinin, precursor 1; encodes substance P, neurokinin A, neuropeptide K, neuropeptide γ
Matrix remodeling	
COL1	Type I procollagen
COL3	Type III procollagen
CYR61	Cysteine rich, angiogenic inducer, 61
DCN	Decorin
MMP1	Matrix metalloproteinase-1
MMP3	Matrix metalloproteinase-3
MMP9	Matrix metalloproteinase-9
Innate immunity	
DEFA1	Defensin, α 1
CXCL12	Chemokine (C-X-C motif) 12
CXCR4	Chemokine (C-X-X motif) receptor type 4
Inflammatory markers	
IL-12B	Interleukin 12B
TNFA	Tumor necrosis factor α

Data from Helfrich YR, Maier LE, Cui Y, et al. Clinical, histologic, and molecular analysis of differences between erythematotelangiectatic rosacea and telangiectatic photoaging. JAMA Dermatol 2015;151(8):825.

into the relationship between rosacea and skin microbes. Recently, in a 2015 genome-wide association study conducted by Chang and colleagues,[12] DNA extraction and genotype analysis was conducted in a discovery group of individuals with greater than 97% European ancestry, composed of 2618 rosacea cases and 20,334 controls. This analysis identified one single-nucleotide polymorphism (SNP), rs763035 found on chromosome 6, that was significantly associated with rosacea in the discovery group and in a replication group of 3205 rosacea cases and 26,262 controls. This SNP was intergenic and located upstream of HLA class II histocompatibility antigen, DR alpha chain (*HLA-DRA*) and downstream of butyrophilin-like 2 (*BTNL2*), which is majorly associated with histocompatibility complex class I. Both genes were connected by coexpression via *HLA-DRB5* and *CIITA* (class II, major histocompatibility complex, transactivator).

Variable expression of HLA-DRA and BTNL2 has been associated with autoimmune diseases with pathologic inflammation, including multiple sclerosis and ulcerative colitis, respectively[12–14] (**Fig. 1**).

Immunohistochemical analysis of papulopustular rosacea skin lesions and analyses for HLA allelic associations with rosacea revealed the presence of HLA-DRA in epidermal Langerhans cells, BTNL2 in keratinocytes, and both genes within perifollicular inflammatory infiltrate and endothelial cells. The staining of endothelial cells for both genes was particularly significant given that vascular dilation and proliferation are cardinal features in rosacea. Further gene association analysis of both the aforementioned discovery and replication groups confirmed the recognition of 3 significant HLA allelic associations of rosacea: *HLA-DRB1*03:01*, *HLA-DQB1*02:01*, and *HLA-DQA1*05:01*. The association of rosacea with these HLA alleles and *HLA-DRA* support the etiologic role of antigen presentation from extracellular sources and, thus, support the connection of various microbes with rosacea[12] (see **Fig. 1**).

Emerging genes of interest, which may be key mediators in skin immune characteristics of rosacea, have been identified in recent studies.[15–17] One such gene target is TRPV4, which encodes for transient receptor potential cation channel subfamily vanilloid member 4 and is activated in keratinocytes in response to UVB light.[16,18] This characteristic of TRPV4 may explain the relationship between rosacea flares and UV exposure.[16,18] In a murine rosacea model, there is upregulation of TRPV4 expression in mast cells in response to LL37, a proteolytic cathelicidin fragment highly expressed in rosacea.[17] The loss of function of TRPV4 leads to the reduction of mast cell degranulation, suggesting that selective inhibition of TRPV4 may be a therapeutic target for rosacea-mediated skin inflammation.

The thymic stromal lymphopoietin (TSLP) gene, a potential therapeutic target of interest, encodes for thymic stromal lymphopoietin, which is a major epithelial cell-derived protein that modulates dendritic cell function in the development of tolerance to commensal microflora in the gut.[15] High expression of TSLP is associated with the decreased activation of dendritic cells and a regular profile of nonpathogenic T-helper 17 (Th17) cells (with a noninflammatory IL-17/IL-10 milieu) in sebaceous gland-rich skin compared with sebaceous gland-poor skin. In PPR, TSLP expression was significantly decreased and associated with an influx of inflammatory dendritic cells and pathogenic Th17 cells with an inflammatory milieu of IL-17 and interferon γ. Linoleic acid exerts increased expression of TSLP, raising into question if the

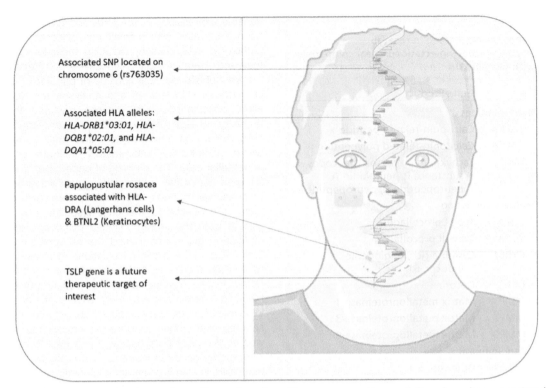

Fig. 1. Rosacea's associated genetic predisposed markers. Numerous genetic associations have been associated with rosacea, most notably rs763035 found on chromosome 6, which is intergenic between *HLA-DRA* and *BTNL2*. TSLP, thymic stromal lymphopoietin. (*From* Servier Medical Art. Available at: http://smart.servier.com/. Under a Creative Commons Attribution 3.0 Unported License. Accessed September 7, 2017.)

altered sebum composition of patients with rosacea may cause a loss of tolerogenic TSLP and lead to the clinical manifestations of PPR (see **Fig. 1**).

Genetic Susceptibility in Familial and Twin Studies

Familial studies of rosacea suggest that genetic factors account for half of the risk of developing rosacea.[9,19] In a cohort study of heterozygous and monozygous twins, monozygous twins demonstrated greater severity of rosacea and a higher correlation with clinical rosacea scores than heterozygous twins.[19] In additional analysis of trait heritability, the genetic contribution to clinical rosacea scores was estimated to be 46%. Common and unique environmental factors, likely UV exposure, age, and microbiome variation, contributed the remaining 54%.

A gain-of-function mutation in the signal transducer and activator of transcription (STAT1) gene associated with rosacea and chronic mucocutaneous candidiasis was noted in a mother and her 3 children.[20] The identified activating mutation of STAT1 (C324R) was associated with early onset rosacea and demodicidosis. The mother had

comorbid autoimmune diseases, including type I diabetes, Sjögren syndrome, hypothyroidism, and celiac disease. All affected family members had thyroid microsomal and antiparietal cell antibodies. These findings suggest there may be an association between the development of autoimmune disorders and the heritability of rosacea.

Genetic Associations with Other Autoimmune Diseases

In continuity with observations of familial rosacea and autoimmune disorders, the association of rosacea with other autoimmune diseases has been confirmed by a population-based case-control study.[21] Rosacea in women was associated with type I diabetes mellitus, multiple sclerosis, and celiac disease.[21] Rosacea in men was associated with rheumatoid arthritis. The recognition of rosacea-associated autoimmune comorbidities may contribute to our understanding of disease genetics and etiopathogenesis.

Rosacea shares several genetic risk loci with autoimmune diseases. The identified HLA allelic associations with rosacea have also been associated with type I diabetes and celiac disease.[12] The haplotype DRB1*03:01-DQB1*02:01-DQA1*05:01

is associated with type I diabetes, and HLA-DRB1*03:01 is associated with retinopathy in type I diabetes. The latter finding may relate to abnormal proliferation of blood vessels observed in ocular manifestations of rosacea (see **Fig. 1**).

HLA-DRA is associated with rosacea and multiple sclerosis; BTNL2 is associated with rosacea, inflammatory bowel disease, and sarcoidosis[12,14,22] (see **Fig. 1**). The shared genetic risk locus with sarcoidosis may relate to the rare granulomatous variant of rosacea, which presents as periocular and centrofacial hard, red, yellow, or brown papules and nodules with progressive scarring.[23] The occurrence of early onset granulomatous rosacea was reported in a female patient with Crohn-associated NOD2/CARD15 polymorphism R702W (arginine to tryptophan).[24] The NOD2/CARD15 gene is also associated with early onset sarcoidosis and is involved in the regulation of NF-kB activation in response to TLR-induced inflammatory stimuli.[25,26] The association between these gene mutations, inflammatory bowel disease, and granulomatous rosacea suggests a role for immune-regulating genes and innate and adaptive immunity in the development of granulomatous diseases.

SUMMARY

There is strong evidence to support the genetic predisposition to rosacea, including a high incidence of familial history, an association with autoimmune disorders, and the identification of associated genetic variants. The theory of evolution of rosacea to induce the production of CAMP for cutaneous pathogenic defense in the absence of UVB-induced ER stress may underscore the role of genetics in the pathogenesis of rosacea. Overlapping and distinct genetic profiles of rosacea subtypes provide the basis for a developmental march across stages of progression of the disease. Yet, the knowledge of the genetic factors at play in the development of rosacea is still very limited. Advancement in our understanding of the genetic component of rosacea is warranted to direct better targeted therapies for improved clinical outcomes.

REFERENCES

1. Elsaie ML, Choudhary S. Updates on the pathophysiology and management of acne rosacea. Postgrad Med 2009;121(5):178–86.
2. Two AM, Wu W, Gallo RL, et al. Rosacea part I. Introduction, categorization, histology, pathogenesis, and risk factors. J Am Acad Dermatol 2015;72(5):749–58.
3. Steinhoff M, Urgen Schauber J, Leyden JJ. New insights into rosacea pathophysiology: a review of recent findings. J Am Acad Dermatol 2013;69(6):S15–26.
4. Holmes AD, Steinhoff M. Integrative concepts of rosacea pathophysiology, clinical presentation and new therapeutics. Exp Dermatol 2017;26(8):659–67.
5. Melnik B. Rosacea: the blessing of the Celts – An approach to pathogenesis through translational research. Acta Derm Venereol 2016;96(2):147–56.
6. Selvaraj P. Vitamin D, vitamin D receptor, and cathelicidin in the treatment of tuberculosis. Vitam Horm 2011;86:307–25.
7. Roby KD, Nardo AD. Innate immunity and the role of the antimicrobial peptide cathelicidin in inflammatory skin disease. Drug Discov Today Dis Mech 2013;10(3–4):e79–82.
8. Chosidow O, Cribier B. Epidemiology of rosacea: updated data. Ann Dermatol Venereol 2011;138:S179–83.
9. Abram K, Silm H, Maaroos H-I, et al. Risk factors associated with rosacea. J Eur Acad Dermatol Venereol 2010;24(5):565–71.
10. Steinhoff M, Buddenkotte J, Aubert J, et al. Clinical, cellular, and molecular aspects in the pathophysiology of rosacea. J Investig Dermatol Symp Proc 2011;15(1):2–11.
11. Helfrich YR, Maier LE, Cui Y, et al. Clinical, histologic, and molecular analysis of differences between erythematotelangiectatic rosacea and telangiectatic photoaging. JAMA Dermatol 2015;151(8):825.
12. Chang ALS, Raber I, Xu J, et al. Assessment of the genetic basis of rosacea by genome-wide association study. J Invest Dermatol 2015;135. https://doi.org/10.1038/jid.2015.53.
13. International Multiple Sclerosis Genetics Consortium, Hafler DA, Compston A, Sawcer S, et al. Risk alleles for multiple sclerosis identified by a genome-wide study. N Engl J Med 2007;357(9):851–62.
14. Anderson CA, Boucher G, Lees CW, et al. Meta-analysis identifies 29 additional ulcerative colitis risk loci, increasing the number of confirmed associations to 47. Nat Genet 2011;43(3):246–52.
15. Dajnoki Z, Béke G, Kapitány A, et al. Sebaceous gland-rich skin is characterized by TSLP expression and distinct immune surveillance which is disturbed in rosacea. J Invest Dermatol 2017;137. https://doi.org/10.1016/j.jid.2016.12.025.
16. Chen Y, Moore CD, Zhang JY, et al. TRPV4 moves toward center-fold in rosacea pathogenesis. J Invest Dermatol 2017;137(4):801–4.
17. Mascarenhas N, Wang Z, Chang Y, et al. TRPV4 mediates mast cell activation in cathelicidin-induced rosacea inflammation. J Invest Dermatol 2017;137:972–5.
18. Moore C, Cevikbas F, Pasolli H, et al. UVB radiation generates sunburn pain and affects skin by activating epidermal TRPV4 ion channels and triggering

endothelin-1 signaling. Proc Natl Acad Sci U S A 2013;110:E3225–34.

19. Aldrich N, Gerstenblith M, Fu P, et al. Genetic vs environmental factors that correlate with rosacea. JAMA Dermatol 2015;151(11):1213.

20. Second J, Korganow A-S, Jannier S, et al. Rosacea and demodicidosis associated with gain-of-function mutation in STAT1. J Eur Acad Dermatol Venereol 2017. https://doi.org/10.1111/jdv.14413.

21. Egeberg A, Hansen PR, Gislason GH, et al. Clustering of autoimmune diseases in patients with rosacea. J Am Acad Dermatol 2016. https://doi.org/10.1016/j.jaad.2015.11.004.

22. Valentonyte R, Hampe J, Huse K, et al. Sarcoidosis is associated with a truncating splice site mutation in BTNL2. Nat Genet 2005;37(4):357–64.

23. Rallis E, Korfitis C. Isotretinoin for the treatment of granulomatous rosacea: case report and review of the literature. J Cutan Med Surg 2012;16(6): 438–41.

24. Van Steensel MAM, Badeloe S, Winnepenninckx V, et al. Granulomatous rosacea and Crohn's disease in a patient homozygous for the Crohn-associated NOD2/CARD15 polymorphism R702W. Exp Dermatol 2008;17(12):1057–8.

25. Watanabe T, Kitani A, Murray PJ, et al. NOD2 is a negative regulator of Toll-like receptor 2-mediated T helper type 1 responses. Nat Immunol 2004;5(8): 800–8.

26. Henckaerts L, Vermeire S. NOD2/CARD15 disease associations other than Crohn's disease. Inflamm Bowel Dis 2007;13(2):235–41.

Validity and Reliability of a Rosacea Self-Assessment Tool

Sara Moradi Tuchayi, MD, MPH[a,*], Hossein Alinia, MD[a],
Lucy Lan, BA[a], Olabola Awosika, MD, MS[a],
Abigail Cline, MD, PhD[b], Leah A. Cardwell, MD[a],
Dennis Hopkinson, MD[a], Irma Richardson, MHA[a],
Karen E. Huang, MS[a], Steven R. Feldman, MD, PhD[a,c,d]

KEYWORDS

- Diagnosis • Disease severity • Erythematotelangiectatic • Papulopustular • Phymatous
- Ocular rosacea • Validity • Reliability

KEY POINTS

- The severity of rosacea in the population is not well characterized.
- The lack of validated tools for measuring rosacea is a major hurdle for obtaining information on rosacea severity.
- A rosacea self-assessment tool (RSAT) was designed to measure the degree of severity of erythematotelangiectatic, papulopustular, phymatous, and ocular rosacea.
- RSAT is a valid and reliable instrument. This tool may facilitate determination of rosacea severity in survey research studies.

INTRODUCTION

Rosacea is a common, chronic skin disorder categorized into 4 subtypes, including erythematotelangiectatic, papulopustular, phymatous, and ocular rosacea.[1] Patients may present with features of 1 or multiple subtypes, and disease severity is highly variable. Despite high clinical referral, physicians lack evidence-based guidelines for rosacea treatments. This may be due to

Disclosure Statement: Moradi Tuchayi, H. Alinia, L. Lan, O. Awosika, A. Cline, L. Cardwell, D. Hopkinson, I. Richardson, and K.E. Huang have no conflicts of interest to disclose. S.R. Feldman is a speaker for Janssen and Taro. He is a consultant and speaker for Galderma, Stiefel/GlaxoSmithKline, Abbott Labs, Leo Pharma Inc. S.R. Feldman has received grants from Galderma, Janssen, Abbott Labs, Amgen, Stiefel, GlaxoSmithKline, Celgene, and Anacor. He is a consultant for Amgen, Baxter, Caremark, Gerson Lehrman Group, Guidepoint Global, Hanall Pharmaceutical Co Ltd, Kikaku, Lilly, Merck & Co Inc, Merz Pharmaceuticals, Mylan, Novartis Pharmaceuticals, Pfizer Inc, Qurient, Suncare Research, and Xenoport. He is on an advisory board for Pfizer Inc. Steven R. Feldman is the founder and holds stock in Causa Research and holds stock and is majority owner in Medical Quality Enhancement Corporation. He receives royalties from UpToDate and Xlibris.
[a] Department of Dermatology, Center for Dermatology Research, Wake Forest University School of Medicine, Medical Center Boulevard, Winston-Salem, NC 27157-1071, USA; [b] Medical College of Georgia, Augusta University, Augusta University Medical Center, 1120 15th Street, Augusta, GA 30912, USA; [c] Department of Pathology, Wake Forest University School of Medicine, Medical Center Boulevard, Winston-Salem, NC 27157-1071, USA; [d] Department of Public Health Sciences, Wake Forest University School of Medicine, Medical Center Boulevard, Winston-Salem, NC 27157-1071, USA
* Corresponding author. Department of Dermatology, Wake Forest University School of Medicine, 4618 Country Club Road, Winston-Salem, NC 27104.
E-mail address: samo_1985@yahoo.com

Dermatol Clin 36 (2018) 93–96
https://doi.org/10.1016/j.det.2017.11.003

the variety of clinical subtypes, the limited understanding of rosacea pathophysiology, or the inconsistent assessment methodologies used in clinical trials.[2] The subjectivity involved in grading the severity of rosacea complicates clinical trials and makes it difficult to assess the efficacy of treatments. Tools used in clinical trials include grading scales, reports of subjective symptoms, and computer analysis of digital photographs.[2–4] These systems allow for a standard method of grading rosacea severity but the variable manifestations of rosacea limit their use.

Physicians must be present to use the grading systems during patient assessment, adding to study expense and requiring patients to regularly return to clinic for evaluation. The use of a validated self-assessment tool would limit cost and maximize convenience. A self-assessment tool is a brief questionnaire that queries patients about rosacea symptoms and severity. Such self-assessments are useful in measuring the degree of depigmentation in vitiligo and the severity of atopic dermatitis.[5,6] Self-assessment instruments allow for closer monitoring of disease status and are an effective means of optimizing communication between patients and physicians. Although a validated self-assessment scale for rosacea erythema severity has been introduced and used in rosacea clinical trials, many rosacea clinical characteristics are not assessed with this measure.[7,8] The aim of this study was to validate a rosacea self-assessment tool (RSAT) to evaluate rosacea severity based on a range of rosacea symptoms characteristic of erythematotelangiectatic, papulopustular, phymatous, and ocular rosacea.

METHODS

A self-assessment tool was designed to measure the degree of erythema (referred to as facial redness), papules (referred to as bumps), pustules (referred to as pimples), rhinophyma (referred to as nose symptoms), and ocular irritation (referred to as eye symptoms) patients experience due to their rosacea. For each measure, 4 pictures with varying degrees of severity (clear to severe) were displayed. Study participants were patients at the Wake Forest Baptist Health dermatology clinic who were diagnosis with rosacea (*International Statistical Classification of Diseases and Related Health Problems*, 9th revision: 695.3). Participants were either new patients, patients returning for follow-up visits, or patients returning for treatments. Participants were asked to complete the questionnaire and then complete it again 30 minutes later. On the same day that the patient completed the RSAT, a physician graded the participant's disease severity using the Investigator Global Severity (IGS) score (**Table 1**). IGS score was used because it allows comparable scoring between the RSAT and the physician assessment. Possible scores included clear (0), almost clear (1), mild (2), moderate (3), and severe (4).

To evaluate gold standard validity, RSAT measurements were compared with IGS scores. The authors evaluated the validity of each of the subcomponents of the RSAT by comparing the erythema, papules, pustules, rhinophyma, and ocular involvement with corresponding averages calculated from the IGS scores. Reliability is the extent to which a test yields the same results on repeated trials, all other things being equal. To assess the reproducibility of participant responses on the RSAT, they completed the RSAT a second time 30 minutes after the first. This time period was chosen to limit bias from a participant's response on the first RSAT and to minimize the changes in severity of the participant's skin lesions.

Pearson correlations were used to assess the relationship between the self-assessment measure and the IGS. Reproducibility of the participant's score was evaluated using an

Table 1
Investigator's global severity score of rosacea

Grade	Score	Clinical Description
Clear	0	No inflammatory lesions present, no erythema, or (at most) very mild erythema
Almost Clear	1	Very mild erythema present, very few small papules or pustules
Mild	2	Mild erythema, several small papules or pustules
Moderate	3	Moderate erythema, several small or large papules or pustules, and up to 2 nodules
Severe	4	Severe erythema, numerous small and/or large papules or pustules may be several nodules

Data from Phase 3 pivotal clinical trial in patients with rosacea. Study No. 0215-R5.C-01–02: A multi-center, investigator-blind clinical trial to assess the safety and efficacy of metronidazole gel, 1% as compared to metronidazole gel vehicle and Noritate cream, 1% in the treatment of rosacea. Dow Pharmaceutical Sciences, 2005. Available at: https://www.accessdata.fda.gov/drugsatfda_docs/nda/2005/021789s000_MetrogelMedR.pdf.

interclass correlation (ICC). Data were managed and analyzed using SAS 9.3 software (SAS Institute Inc, Cary, NC, USA).

RESULTS

A total of 46 participants completed the self-assessment. Most participants were female gender (70%, n = 32) and white (91%, n = 42). Two participants were African American (4%), 1 was Asian (2%), and 1 identified as multiracial (2%). Of these, 82% (n = 37) considered themselves fair-skinned.

Self-Report Scoring

The median self-reported scores were 2 (interquartile range [IQR]: 1,2) for redness, 1 (IQR: 1,2) for bumps and pimples, 1 (IQR: 1,2) for rhinophyma, and 1 (IQR: 1,2) for ocular involvement. The median IGS score was 2 (IQR: 2,3). There was moderate correlation among self-reported redness, rhinophyma, or the sum of redness and bumps or pimples and the IGS (**Table 2**). Using linear regression, the redness and bumps or pimples combined score significantly regressed against the IGS (P = .03).

Test–Retest Reliability

All 46 participants completed the second RSAT. All items had acceptable ICCs: redness (ICC = 0.75), bumps (ICC = 0.83), rhinophyma (ICC = 0.88), and ocular (ICC = 0.87). The authors also assessed if the retest summed score of the redness and bumps or pimples was consistently correlated with the IGS. Using linear regression, IGS was similarly associated with this second measurement (slope = 0.47, P = .003, multivariate coefficient [R^2] = 0.10). Test–retest RSAT measurements were correlated.

Table 2
Correlation of each self-reported measure to the investigator global severity score

Self-Reported Item	Pearson Correlation	P-Value
Redness	0.31	.04
Bumps	0.20	.18
Rhinophyma	0.44	.003
Ocular involvement	0.01	.92
Sum of redness and bumps score	0.32	.03

DISCUSSION

The self-assessment of redness and rhinophyma demonstrated moderate correlation with the IGS score, and the redness and bumps or pimples combined score demonstrated significant regression against the IGS score. There was also consistency between the test–retest, with ICC measuring between 0.75 and 0.88. These correlations suggest that the self-assessment tool could be used for accurate and reliable assessment of erythema and rhinophyma in rosacea patients. The correlation between the RSAT score and the IGS score observed in this sample suggests that the RSAT would be well-suited for large populations.

RSAT holds promise in enabling patients to objectively assess their rosacea severity. Compared against the IGS scores, Pearson correlation ranged from 0.20 to 0.44. Whether other graded scales of rosacea severity would provide a closer correlation remains to be investigated. Similar self-assessment validity studies in dermatology include the Self-Assessed Vitiligo Area Scoring Index (SAVASI), the Patient-Oriented SCORing Atopic Dermatitis (PO-SCORAD), and the Patient's Self-Assessment (PSA) scale.[5,6,9] The PSA scale captures patients' self-assessment of erythema associated with rosacea. It has been used in clinical studies to evaluate the efficacy of brimonidine tartrate gel for the treatment of facial erythema of rosacea.[7,9] However, the variety of rosacea clinical characteristics necessitates the use of a scale that assesses a range of symptoms. In addition to measuring erythema, the RSAT also measures the severity of papules or pustules, rhinophyma, and ocular irritation. The use of pictures allows patients to accurately compare their symptoms with standardized photographs. This enables patients to understand the severity of their symptoms in comparison to the progression of rosacea.

There was correlation between the RSAT and IGS across the broad spectrum of clinical manifestations of rosacea, despite the limited range of scores in this population; few patients were classified as 0 (clear) or 4 (severe). This was a single-center study and most of the study participants were female gender and white, which may have limited generalizability of the data. Further validation in a more diverse population with a wider range of severity would likely provide greater correlation between the RSAT and the IGS. This self-assessment tool represents a valuable instrument for assessing rosacea severity in large-scale clinical trials. It may also have utility in providing a simple quantitative measure of rosacea severity in clinical practice.

REFERENCES

1. Powell FC. Rosacea. N Engl J Med 2005;352:793–803. Available at: http://www.ncbi.nlm.nih.gov/pubmed/15728812. Accessed Sep 5, 2017.

2. Hopkinson D, Moradi Tuchayi S, Alinia H, et al. Assessment of rosacea severity: a review of evaluation methods used in clinical trials. J Am Acad Dermatol 2015;73:138–43.e4. Available at: http://linkinghub.elsevier.com/retrieve/pii/S0190962215013614. Accessed Sep 5, 2017.

3. Bamford JT. Interobserver variation in the assessment of rosacea. Arch Dermatol 1998;134:508. Available at: http://www.ncbi.nlm.nih.gov/pubmed/9554308. Accessed Sep 5, 2017.

4. Wilkin J, Dahl M, Detmar M, et al. Standard grading system for rosacea: report of the National Rosacea Society Expert Committee on the classification and staging of rosacea. J Am Acad Dermatol 2004;50:907–12. Available at: http://linkinghub.elsevier.com/retrieve/pii/S0190962204005353. Accessed Sep 5, 2017.

5. Komen L, van der Kraaij GE, van der Veen JPW, et al. The validity, reliability and acceptability of the SAVASI; a new self-assessment score in vitiligo. J Eur Acad Dermatol Venereol 2015;29:2145–51. Available from: http://doi.wiley.com/10.1111/jdv.13161. Accessed Sep 5, 2017.

6. Stalder JF, Barbarot S, Wollenberg A, et al. Patient-Oriented SCORAD (PO-SCORAD): a new self-assessment scale in atopic dermatitis validated in Europe. Allergy 2011;66:1114–21. Available from: http://doi.wiley.com/10.1111/j.1398-9995.2011.02577.x. Accessed Sep 5, 2017.

7. Fowler J, Tan J, Jackson JM, et al. Treatment of facial erythema in patients with rosacea with topical brimonidine tartrate: correlation of patient satisfaction with standard clinical endpoints of improvement of facial erythema. J Eur Acad Dermatol Venereol 2015;29:474–81. Available from: http://doi.wiley.com/10.1111/jdv.12587. Accessed Sep 5, 2017.

8. Fowler J, Jarratt M, Moore A, et al. Once-daily topical brimonidine tartrate gel 0·5% is a novel treatment for moderate to severe facial erythema of rosacea: results of two multicentre, randomized and vehicle-controlled studies. Br J Dermatol 2012;166:633–41. Available from: http://doi.wiley.com/10.1111/j.1365-2133.2011.10716.x. Accessed Sep 5, 2017.

9. Tan J, Leoni M. Erythema of rosacea: validation of patient's self-assessment grading scale. J Drugs Dermatol 2015;14:841–4. Available from: http://www.ncbi.nlm.nih.gov/pubmed/26267728. Accessed Sep 5, 2017.

Measurement of Disease Severity in a Population of Rosacea Patients

Hossein Alinia, MD[a], Sara Moradi Tuchayi, MD, MPH[a],
Sara M. James, BS[a], Leah A. Cardwell, MD[a],*,
Sonali Nanda, MS[a], Naeim Bahrami, PhD[a,b],
Olabola Awosika, MD, MS[c], Irma Richardson, MHA[a],
Karen E. Huang, MS[a], Steven R. Feldman, MD, PhD[a,d,e]

KEYWORDS

- Epidemiology • Rosacea • Severity • Self-assessment • Survey • Papulopustular
- Erythematotelangectatic • Demographics

KEY POINTS

- The authors developed a validated self-assessment tool that facilitates more accurate assessment of rosacea severity in survey studies.
- Prior to this assessment tool, determination of rosacea severity was based on costly in-person clinic visits.
- Rosacea was more severe in men and younger patients; age significantly predicted disease severity, with younger patients (age<60 years) reporting more severe rosacea.
- Younger patients also spent longer taking care of their rosacea on a daily basis, which may increase the morbidity of the disease.

Disclosure Statement: Dr S.R. Feldman is a speaker for Janssen and Taro. He is a consultant and speaker for Galderma, Stiefel, GlaxoSmithKline, Abbott Labs, and Leo Pharma Inc. Dr S.R. Feldman has received grants from Galderma, Janssen, Abbott Labs, Amgen, Stiefel, GlaxoSmithKline, Celgene, and Anacor. He is a consultant for Amgen, Baxter, Caremark, Gerson Lehrman Group, Guidepoint Global, Hanall Pharmaceutical Co Ltd, Kikaku, Lilly, Merck & Co Inc, Merz Pharmaceuticals, Mylan, Novartis Pharmaceuticals, Pfizer Inc, Qurient, Suncare Research, and Xenoport. He is on an advisory board for Pfizer Inc. Dr S.R. Feldman is the founder and holds stock in Causa Research and holds stock and is majority owner in Medical Quality Enhancement Corporation. He receives Royalties from UpToDate and Xlibris. H. Alinia, S.M. Tuchayi, S. James, L. Cardwell, S. Nanda, I. Richardson, K. Huang, O. Awosika, and N. Bahrami have no conflicts to disclose.
[a] Department of Dermatology, Center for Dermatology Research, Wake Forest School of Medicine, Medical Center Boulevard, Winston-Salem, NC 27157-1071, USA; [b] Department of Biomedical Engineering, Virginia Polytechnic Institute and State University-Wake Forest University, Medical Center Boulevard, Winston-Salem, NC 27157-1071, USA; [c] Department of Dermatology, The George Washington Medical Faculty Associates, 2150 Pennsylvania Avenue NorthWest, 2B-427, Washington, DC 20037, USA; [d] Department of Pathology, Wake Forest School of Medicine, Medical Center Boulevard, Winston-Salem, NC 27157-1071, USA; [e] Department of Public Health Sciences, Wake Forest School of Medicine, Medical Center Boulevard, Winston-Salem, NC 27157-1071, USA
* Corresponding author. Department of Dermatology, Wake Forest School of Medicine, Medical Center Boulevard, Winston-Salem, NC 27157-1071.
E-mail address: lcardwell06@gmail.com

Dermatol Clin 36 (2018) 97–102
https://doi.org/10.1016/j.det.2017.11.004

derm.theclinics.com

INTRODUCTION

Rosacea is a chronic skin disorder with unclear pathogenesis. The National Rosacea Society Expert Committee created a grading system and identified 4 subtypes: erythematotelangiectatic, papulopustular, phymatous, and ocular.[1] Much remains unknown about the natural history of rosacea; it is unclear if each subtype is a discrete form of disease or if there is a natural progression between subtypes.[2] Rosacea may progress from the erythematotelangiectatic to the papulopustular subtype, with a majority of patients developing the papulopustular subtype prior to phymatous changes.[3] Longstanding, untreated rosacea can progress to phymatous changes, fibrosis, and disfigurement.[2]

The estimated prevalence of rosacea ranges from less than 1% to greater than 20%.[4–8] Previous epidemiologic studies have provided few answers about the severity of rosacea and its relation to patients' demographics within populations because there is a paucity of validated severity measures.[9]

The authors developed a validated self-assessment tool that facilitates more accurate assessment of rosacea severity in survey studies (Tuchayi SM, Alinia H, Lan L, et al. Validity and reliability of a rosacea self-assessment tool. Submitted for publication). Prior to this assessment tool, determination of rosacea severity was based on costly in-person clinic visits. The purpose of this study is to report the distribution of self-assessed rosacea severity scores within a population of rosacea patients and describe the relationship between disease severity and demographic factors.

METHODS

Subjects were adult patients at the Wake Forest Baptist Medical Center dermatology clinic from 2011 to 2014 who received a clinical diagnosis of rosacea (*International Classification of Disease, Ninth Revision*, code: 695.3) from a Wake Forest dermatologist. Institutional Review Board approval was obtained prior to initiation of this study. Data were collected from October 2014 until February 2015. Eligible rosacea patients were identified using the Wake Forest Baptist Hospital transitional data warehouse and the electronic medical record system. Children were excluded because rosacea is not typically present in children and the measures used were not validated in children.

To recruit subjects to complete the survey in person, 165 patients were contacted via phone. A total of 46 subjects who came to the office for the validation of self-assessment tool study were recruited to complete the survey during the same visit. A pre-survey letter was mailed to 432 subjects to inform them that they would receive the survey via mail. Twenty subjects declined to receive the survey. Surveys were mailed to 412 subjects. Sixteen surveys were returned by the post office because of address changes. A total of 195 surveys (149 via mail and 46 in person) were completed and analyzed (**Fig. 1**). All participants who completed the survey by mail also completed a previously validated self-assessment tool. Patients selected images to identify the severity of their symptoms; categories included erythema, papulopustular lesions, ocular symptoms, and nasal involvement. Scores ranged from 2 (least severe) to 8 (most severe). Subjects were offered financial compensation for their travel expenses and time. The overall response rate of the survey was 44.1%.

Results were reported using descriptive statistics. Regression analysis was performed to identify independent outcome predictors. To study the relationship between age and demographic variables, the population was divided into two groups: ages greater than or equal to 60 years and ages less than 60 years. Correlation of variables with duration of disease was also studied by creating two groups: duration of disease greater than or equal to 11 years and duration less than 11 years. Between-groups comparisons were completed using chi-square tests for proportions and t tests or analysis of variance for continuous variables.

The results of the survey were compared with 4 studies:

Feldman and colleagues (2001)[10]: a database analysis of the US National Ambulatory Medical Care Survey from 1990 to 1997 querying office visits associated with the diagnosis of rosacea.

Spoendlin and colleagues (2012)[11]: a retrospective case-control study of 60,042 patients with rosacea in the United Kingdom using the UK-based General Practice Research Database.

Kyriakis and colleagues (2005)[12]: a cross-sectional study of 615 rosacea patients from 1995 to 2002 in an outpatient population at a state hospital dermatology clinic in Greece.

Khaled and colleagues (2010)[13]: a retrospective study of 244 rosacea patients diagnosed in the outpatient Dermatology Department of the Charles Nicolle Hospital in Tunisia between 1990 and 2003.

RESULTS

Responders Versus Nonresponders

Nonresponders consisted of 263 patients (44.1%) who received phone calls, the mail

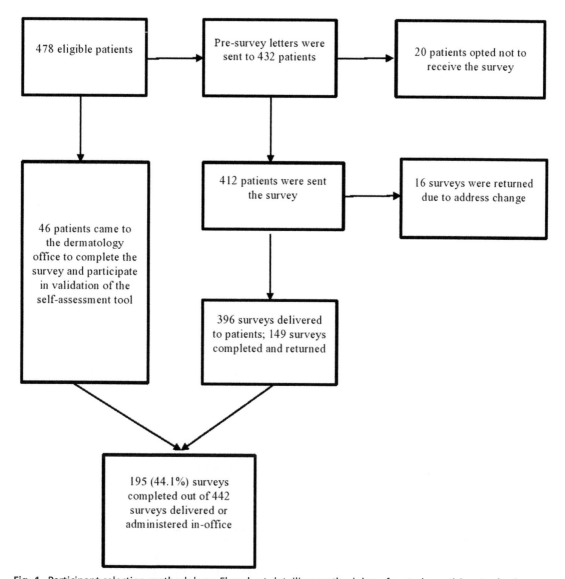

Fig. 1. Participant selection methodology. Flowchart detailing methodology for study participant selection.

survey, or both; this number includes 16 patients who changed their address. Similar to responders, average age of nonresponders was 56.9 years and 64.2% (n = 169) of nonresponders were women.

Demographic Variables

The mean age of survey responders was 58 years ± 13 (mean ± SD), with a range of 20 years to 87 years of age. In Feldman and colleagues' study,[10] mean age was 50 ± 17 years (mean ±SD), whereas in Kyriakis and colleagues'[12] study the median age was 48 years in women and 59 years in men. The age distribution of the authors' study population was similar to

that of the Kyriakis and colleagues'[12] study (Fig. 2).

The authors' sample consisted of more women (n = 155; 81.2%) than men (n = 36; 18.8%). Similar to the authors' study, Spoendlin and colleagues,[11] Feldman and colleagues,[10] and Khaled and colleagues[13] reported that more women than men have rosacea (62%, 69%, and 71%, respectively). Conversely, in Kyriakis and colleagues'[12] study, both genders were equally represented (relative prevalence 1.22%). Only one other study has reported an equal prevalence across genders.[14]

The average duration of disease was 11.5 ± 10.5 years (mean ±SD), with a range of 3 months to 58 years. A majority of participants were white (95.3%), with responders from several

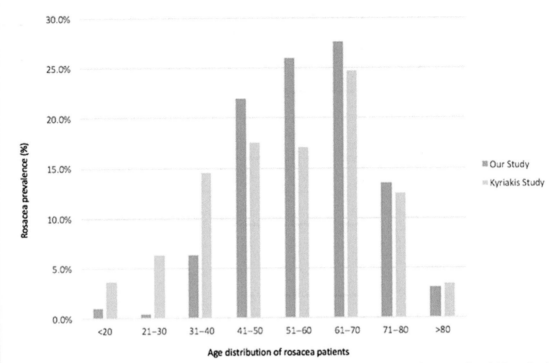

Fig. 2. Rosacea prevalence. Prevalence of rosacea by age in the authors' study population and Kyriakis and colleagues'[12] study. The distribution of rosacea prevalence in our study was similar to Kyriakis and colleagues'[12] study. Rosacea had the highest prevalence in middle-aged patients in both studies.

other racial groups, including African American (2.1%), Hispanic (1.6%), and less than 1% each of Asian and other races.

Severity

A majority of patients had severity scores between 2 and 4 out of 8 (most severe) (**Fig. 3**). Eye symptoms were reported in a higher proportion of patients (n = 165; 86.4%) than in Spoendlin and colleagues'[11] population (n = 12,480; 20.8%).

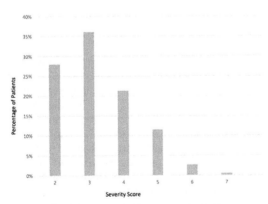

Fig. 3. Distribution of self-assessment severity scores. Depicts self-selected severity scores using a previously validated self-assessment tool. Most patients reported mild to moderate rosacea.

Most participants reported mild nasal involvement (n = 139, 75.5%); others reported moderate nasal involvement (n = 42; 22.8%) and severe nasal involvement (n = 3; 1.6%). No patient reported very severe nasal involvement. Nasal involvement was more likely in men (39%) than in women (20%; $P = .03$). The low prevalence and male preponderance of severe and very severe nasal involvement agrees with prior studies. Rhinophyma was reported in 0.7% (n = 822) of cases in Spoendlin and colleagues'[11] study, with 80.3% being men, and in 0.02% (n = 14) of patients in Kyriakis and colleagues'[12] study, with 71.2% being men.

Rosacea Treatment

Average daily time spent taking care of rosacea was 5 minutes (median), with a range of 0 to 120 minutes. A total of 184 participants (96.3%) had not treated their rosacea with surgery. Three subjects had undergone surgery, and 4 subjects had been treated with electrocautery. Light therapy was used by 19.9% of responders.

Demographic Correlation with Severity

Age and disease severity were negatively correlated (r = −0.19; $P = .01$). Self-assessment severity scores were significantly higher in participants less than 60 years old (mean 3.43 ± 1.07) compared with those age 60 years or greater (mean 3.09 ± 1.13; $P = .04$). Participants younger than 60 years reported spending an average of 5 minutes (median with a range of 0–120 minutes) managing their rosacea symptoms versus 5 minutes (median with a range of 0–40 minutes) in those greater than 60 years old ($P = .01$). Age did not predict presence of eye symptoms ($P = .53$), nasal involvement ($P = .39$), or use of light therapy ($P = .72$).

Self-assessment severity scores were significantly higher in men (3.6 ± 1.3) than women (3.2 ± 1.0; $P = .04$). Gender was not significantly correlated with time spent taking care of rosacea ($P = .38$), use of light therapy ($P = .82$), or presence of eye symptoms ($P = .11$).

Duration of disease was not significantly related to disease severity ($P = .62$). There was also no correlation between disease duration and self-assessment severity score ($P = .19$), presence of eye symptoms ($P<.999$), nasal involvement ($P = .58$), use of light therapy ($P = .73$), or daily time spent taking care of rosacea symptoms ($P = .14$).

Comorbidities

Twenty participants (10.5%) reported chronic migraines/headaches, 60 (31.4%) reported high blood pressure, 25 (13.1%) reported depression, and 25 (13.1%) reported anxiety (**Table 1**). Khaled and colleagues[13] reported comorbid diseases in 54 of 244 patients (22.1%), with diabetes (n = 13) and hypertension (n = 10) most often

Table 1
Comorbid medical diseases

Disease	Frequency (n = 194)
Hypertension	60 (30.9%)
Depression	26 (13.4%)
Anxiety[a]	25 (13.0%)
Chronic headaches/migraines	21 (10.8%)
Cancer	15 (7.7%)
Thyroid disease	7 (3.6%)
Diabetes	7 (3.6%)
Kidney disease	6 (3.1%)
Heart valve disease	4 (2.1%)
Chronic obstructive pulmonary disease	4 (2.1%)

Patient-reported comorbid medical diseases.
[a] n = 193 for anxiety.

Table 2
Coexisting skin diseases

Condition	Frequency (n = 194)
Acne	76 (39.2%)
Skin allergy	27 (13.9%)
Psoriasis	21 (10.8%)
Atopic dermatitis	44 (22.7%)
Seborrheic dermatitis	21 (10.8%)
Melanoma	11 (5.7%)
Nonmelanoma skin cancer[a]	38 (19.7%)

Patient-reported coexisting skin diseases.
[a] n = 193 for nonmelanoma skin cancer.

reported. Patients in the authors' study also frequently had a history of other skin diseases (**Table 2**).

DISCUSSION

Rosacea was more severe in men and younger patients. The authors' study population correlated well with other rosacea epidemiology studies, but ocular symptoms were reported in a higher percentage of patients.[11] Age significantly predicted disease severity, with younger patients (age <60 years) reporting more severe rosacea. Younger patients also spent longer taking care of their rosacea on a daily basis, which may increase the morbidity of the disease. Little is known about the biological relationship between patient age and rosacea severity. Younger patients or patients with more severe disease may have been more likely to fill out the survey. Conversely, the authors' finding of more severe disease in younger patients may indicate that either more severe rosacea presents earlier or that rosacea improves with age. Based on the theory that rosacea progresses with time, the authors' results suggest that severe rosacea presents earlier.[3] The pathophysiology of rosacea is poorly understood, but future studies may investigate whether the biology of rosacea, such as chemokine levels, differs based on patient age.

There are several limitations to the authors' study. The study population consists of university dermatology clinic patients who may not be representative of patients in the general population. The authors' hospital system, however, does not require referrals and cares for a large percentage of the surrounding community. Although only 44.1% of patients responded to the survey, nonresponders matched responders for age and gender.

Participants of this study had a high rate of self-reported comorbid conditions, specifically hypertension, chronic headaches/migraines, depression, and anxiety. The increased prevalence of depression and anxiety corroborates findings of prior studies.[15] The odds ratio for depression in rosacea patients is 4.81 (95% CI, 1.39–16.62).[16] High rates of anxiety and depression may contribute to increased health care costs for rosacea patients, because they have more general practitioner visits than patients without rosacea.[11]

This study used a reliable and validated patient self-assessment tool to show that rosacea is more severe in younger patients and men. This relationship between disease severity and demographics is important to consider when treating and studying rosacea.

REFERENCES

1. Wilkin J, Dahl M, Detmar M, et al. Standard grading system for rosacea: report of the national rosacea society expert committee on the classification and staging of rosacea. J Am Acad Dermatol 2004; 50(6):907–12.
2. Steinhoff M, Schauber J, Leyden JJ. New insights into rosacea pathophysiology: a review of recent findings. J Am Acad Dermatol 2013;69(6 Suppl 1): S15–26.
3. Tan J, Blume-Peytavi U, Ortonne JP, et al. An observational cross-sectional survey of rosacea: clinical associations and progression between subtypes. Br J Dermatol 2013;169(3):555–62.
4. Lomholt G. Prevalence of skin diseases in a population; a census study from the Faroe Islands. Dan Med Bull 1964;11:1–7.
5. Augustin M, Herberger K, Hintzen S, et al. Prevalence of skin lesions and need for treatment in a cohort of 90,880 workers. Br J Dermatol 2011; 165(4):865–73.
6. Schaefer I, Rustenbach SJ, Zimmer L, et al. Prevalence of skin diseases in a cohort of 48,665 employees in Germany. Dermatology 2008;217(2): 169–72.
7. Abram K, Silm H, Oona M. Prevalence of rosacea in an Estonian working population using a standard classification. Acta Derm Venereol 2010;90(3): 269–73.
8. Moustafa F, Hopkinson D, Huang KE, et al. Prevalence of rosacea in community settings. J Cutan Med Surg 2015;19(2):149–52.
9. Hopkinson D, Moradi Tuchayi S, Alinia H, et al. Assessment of rosacea severity: A review of evaluation methods used in clinical trials. J Am Acad Dermatol 2015;73(1):138–43.
10. Feldman SR, Hollar CB, Gupta AK, et al. Women commonly seek care for rosacea: Dermatologists frequently provide the care. Cutis 2001;68(2): 156–60.
11. Spoendlin J, Voegel JJ, Jick SS, et al. A study on the epidemiology of rosacea in the U.K. Br J Dermatol 2012;167(3):598–605.
12. Kyriakis KP, Palamaras I, Terzoudi S, et al. Epidemiologic aspects of rosacea. J Am Acad Dermatol 2005;53(5):918–9.
13. Khaled A, Hammami H, Zeglaoui F, et al. Rosacea: 244 tunisian cases. Tunis Med 2010;88(8):597–601.
14. Marks R. The enigma of rosacea. J Dermatolog Treat 2007;18(6):326–8.
15. Chodkiewicz J, Salamon M, Miniszewska J, et al. Psychosocial impact of rosacea. Przegl Lek 2007; 64(12):997–1001.
16. Gupta MA, Gupta AK, Chen SJ, et al. Comorbidity of rosacea and depression: an analysis of the National Ambulatory Medical Care Survey and National Hospital Ambulatory Care Survey–outpatient department data collected by the U.S. National Center for Health Statistics from 1995 to 2002. Br J Dermatol 2005;153(6):1176–81.

Psychosocial Burden and Other Impacts of Rosacea on Patients' Quality of Life

Elias Oussedik, BSc[a],*, Marc Bourcier, MD[b], Jerry Tan, MD[c,d]

KEYWORDS

- Stigmatization • Dermatology Life Quality Index • Depression • Social anxiety
- Psychiatric comorbidity • Chronic disease • RosaQoL • Outcome measures

KEY POINTS

- Rosacea has a major impact on quality of life and self-esteem.
- Stigmatization, depression, social anxiety, and other psychiatric comorbidities are common in rosacea patients.
- Pharmacologic interventions that improve disease severity seem to concurrently improve quality of life.

INTRODUCTION

Rosacea is a common and chronic skin disorder characterized by persistent redness on the convex surfaces of the face in addition to a spectrum of facial clinical features including flushing, papules, pustules, telangiectases, phyma, and ocular involvement.[1] Estimated prevalence ranges from 0.1% to 22%[2–5]; however, it is thought that many cases of rosacea are undiagnosed.[5,6] Recently, a validated screening instrument to facilitate population screening for rosacea (Rosascreen)[7] has been developed. Using this tool, rosacea's estimated prevalence in Russia and Germany has been reported at 5% and 12%, respectively.[5]

Physical appearance and facial features affect a wide variety of essential social outcomes, including hiring decisions, relationships, and selection of mates.[8] Facial characteristics are also critical in influencing how others perceive attractiveness.[8–10] Tabloids, television shows, and movies are all filled with attractive faces characterized by facial symmetry, averageness, sexual characteristics, skin health, and color.[8] Redness, flushing, papules, pustules, and phyma all negatively affect the skin health and color paradigm of attractiveness and, therefore, may lead to negative social outcomes.[11] In humans, facial flushing may suggest confrontation and anger, embarrassment, or excessive alcohol intake, all of which signal negative traits and may confer stigmatization.[12,13]

Rosacea is often noticeable by others, most notably for persistent facial redness, which often leads to an assortment of social and emotional

Disclosure Statement: E. Oussedik is a consultant for Galderma. M. Bourcier is an investigator advisory board member, and consultant for AbbVie, Amgen, Celgene, Eli-Lilly, Janssen, Leo Pharma, Novartis, Pfizer, and UCB. J. Tan has been an advisor, consultant, speaker, and/or clinical investigator for Allergan, Cipher, Dermira, Galderma, Roche, Stiefel GSK, and Valeant.

a Center for Dermatology Research, Department of Dermatology, Wake Forest School of Medicine, Medical Center Boulevard, Winston-Salem, NC 27157-1071, USA; b Hop G. L. Dumont, Dermatology, Dermatology Clinic, 35 Providence Street, Moncton, New Brunswick E1C 8X3, Canada; c Schulich School of Medicine and Dentistry, Western University, Windsor Campus, Medical Education Building, 401 Sunset Avenue, Windsor, Ontario N9B3P4, Canada; d Windsor Clinical Research Inc, 2224 Walker Road, Suite 300B, Windsor, Ontario N8W 5L7, Canada
* Corresponding author.
E-mail address: Elias.Oussedik@gmail.com

Dermatol Clin 36 (2018) 103–113
https://doi.org/10.1016/j.det.2017.11.005

derm.theclinics.com

consequences.[14] Social anxiety, stigmatization, depression, phobia, and even psychiatric comorbidities are commonly present alongside rosacea. Many studies have revealed an adverse impact in health-related quality of life (HRQoL) in rosacea patients.[13,15] Therefore, an understanding of the instruments available in measuring quality of life (QoL) is important. Such tools may be used to delineate whether certain therapies are more effective than others in decreasing rosacea's psychosocial impact. The objective of this article is to provide a clinical perspective on rosacea's psychosocial implication on patient QoL, focusing on rosacea's psychological, social, and occupational impact.

Quality of Life and Burden of Disease

QoL involves a multitude of domains centered on an individual's wellbeing, mainly encompassing a physical, psychological, social, sexual, and occupational perspective.[16] For example, QoL determinants within rosacea include: (1) physical factors such as pain, irritation, burning sensation, dryness, and ocular symptoms[17,18]; (2) psychosocial factors such as anger, depression, lowered self-esteem, stigmatization, worry, embarrassment, social phobia, anxiety, or frustration[15,19–21]; and (3) occupational factors such as days lost from work, decreased job opportunities, or pharmacoeconomic considerations.[19,22] However, the understanding of rosacea's sexual impact is limited and still nascent.[21] During concept elicitation in the development of a rosacea-specific QoL instrument, rosacea's impact on sexuality was not weighted highly by patients, and the sex domain was later deleted from the QoL instrument as an insensitive item.[23]

PSYCHOSOCIAL IMPACT OF ROSACEA

Rosacea's clinical severity does not correlate with its psychosocial severity because very mild cases may sometimes be accompanied by severe psychosocial impact.[24] This may be due to the facial localization of rosacea, making it difficult to conceal.[25] In a survey conducted by the National Rosacea Society involving more than 400 rosacea subjects, 75% shared feelings of low self-esteem, 70% embarrassment, 69% frustration, and 56% thought they had been robbed of their pleasure or happiness.[26]

Stigmatization

Stigmatized individuals with rosacea are affected more greatly by others' response to their disease than the disease itself.[13,27,28] Those with rosacea often share the perception that they are the object of ridicule and the recipients of discourteous comments.[29,30] Among 807 adult patients with rosacea, in France, Germany, the United States, and the United Kingdom who completed an online survey, one-third reported feelings of stigmatization.[13] Male patients are more adversely affected by stigmatization.[13] This finding correlates with other rosacea studies in which men tend to experience more severe signs and symptoms (phenotypes) relating to their rosacea than women.[31,32] Those who experience stigmatization due to their rosacea have a higher rate of depression (36.7% vs 21.1%) and are more inclined to avoid social situations (54.2% vs 2.0%).[13]

In an online survey of more than 5000 unaffected participants shown images of faces with and without erythema, the images with facial redness were perceived as being less relaxed, less healthy, and less well.[21] Facial redness was strongly associated with perceptions of poor health and negative personality traits.[21]

Although other studies in dermatology have explored the levels of stigmatization between skin diseases, with psoriasis being among the most highly stigmatized skin conditions,[33] no studies to date have included rosacea among the comparators. In a cohort of 168 German subjects with rosacea, rejection scores using the Questionnaire on Experience with Skin Complaints were significantly higher than the reported scores in an independent sample of individuals with psoriasis and atopic dermatis.[34]

Psychosocial Comorbidities

Rosacea is associated with multiple comorbidities.[35–38] The most common associated psychosocial comorbidities include depression, social anxiety, and social phobia.[24] Social anxiety and social phobia lead to stress, which may physiologically exacerbate facial redness due to the release of proinflammatory agents.[39–41] Environmental stressors induce and generate matrix metalloproteinases, reactive oxygen species, toll-like receptor signaling, and neuropeptides, which modulate the expression of chemokines and cytokines, further activating the immune system.[42] Selective serotonin reuptake inhibitors, which are considered first-line therapy for major depressive disorder, have some evidence of efficacy in the treatment of the flushing associated with rosacea.[43,44] However, depression or other affective disorders are not considered primary etiologic factors for the development of rosacea.[45]

Depression and social anxiety
Depression is common among rosacea presents, with approximately 32% experiencing some levels

of depression.[20] In a cohort of 184 subjects in the United States with rosacea who completed the Patient Health Questionnaire-9, 21.8% had minimal depressive symptoms, 7.1% had minor depression, 1.0% had moderate major depression, and 1.0% had severe major depression.[46] There was a statistically significant direct relationship between rosacea severity and depression severity, more severe rosacea was associated with more severe depression. Similarly, in a Danish nationwide cohort study of 4,632,341 individuals with a clinical diagnosis of rosacea and depression, there was a rosacea severity-dependent increased risk of developing depression.[47] Younger patients and those with a low socioeconomic status were at increased risk of developing depression.[47] Other studies have also delineated the increased rate of depression in rosacea patients. An analysis of the National Ambulatory Medical Care Survey and National Hospital Ambulatory Care Survey revealed that 65.1% of rosacea patients diagnosed with a comorbid psychiatric illness had a clinical diagnosis of depression, higher than the 29.9% prevalence of depression among all psychiatric visits in the United States between 1995 and 2002.[36]

In a metaanalysis using the EuroQoL 5-dimension (EQ-5D)[26] questionnaire in 1624 rosacea subjects, 26.4% of subjects reported being moderately or extremely anxious or depressed and cited comorbid anxiety and depression as the main reasons for decreased HRQoL.[22] In a National Rosacea Society survey of 1675 rosacea subjects, 54% shared feelings of anxiety, 43% of depression, and 52% of social phobia (purposely avoiding face-to-face social contact).[19] In a survey conducted by the National Rosacea Society, nearly one-third of respondents felt uncomfortable when dating due to their facial erythema.[21]

Although rosacea and depression are traditionally considered 2 distinct diseases, both share similar inflammatory pathways.[48–51] Shared mediators include interleukin (IL)-1, IL-12, and IL-17, among others.[42,52–54] Such a finding raises the hypothesis that depression in rosacea may be ascribed to elevated proinflammatory cytokines and not solely secondary to rosacea's psychosocial impact. Further studies delineating this possible association are warranted.

Occupational Impact

The mean annual management cost of rosacea in the United States is $347, with a medical cost of $56 and a pharmacy cost of $291 (based on 2013 US dollar estimates).[24] The impact of rosacea also extends to the workplace, where 50% of patients have purposely missed work because of the psychosocial impact of their condition.[19] Using the Productivity and Social Life Questionnaire, 8.3% of 993 rosacea patients with mild-to-moderate symptoms felt that their work productivity was negatively affected by their condition.[22] In patients with severe rosacea-associated facial redness, 47.8% cited that facial redness interfered with their work life.[22]

Rosacea may also hinder patients from obtaining employment. In the same study in which images of individuals with facial redness were perceived as being less relaxed, less healthy, and less well, they were also perceived as being less likely to be hired for a job.[21]

TOOLS TO MEASURE QUALITY OF LIFE

Measuring the objective therapeutic effects of different treatment options in rosacea can be difficult because there are few validated, standardized clinical or research tools to measure its signs and symptoms.[55,56] Traditionally, clinical investigators have placed greater emphasis on participant-reported improvements, physician global assessments of improvement, assessments of erythema and/or telangiectasia, and/or papule and pustule count.[55] However, these clinical measures often correlate poorly with QoL.[23,57] Many clinicians and regulatory authorities have recognized the importance of assessing QoL and including it as an outcome measure in clinical trials.[22,58] The Cochrane Review of interventions for rosacea considered the change in HRQoL to be the most important patient-centered outcome measure in clinical trials.[58] In the ROSacea COnsensus recommendations, panelists unanimously agreed that a tool measuring the QoL impact of rosacea is of critical importance.[59]

HRQoL measures exist at 3 different levels, with each demonstrating differing echelons of sensitivity in assessing QoL (Table 1). There are: (1) generic HRQoL measures, (2) disease class–specific HRQoL measures, and (3) disease-specific HRQoL measures. Generic HRQoL measures are less sensitive to disease class–specific or disease-specific measures of QoL because they assess QoL without direct reference to the signs or symptoms of a specific class of disease. Popular disease class–specific HRQoL measures used in dermatology include measures such as the Dermatology Life Quality Index (DLQI)[60] and Skindex-29.[57] Although these dermatology-specific measures are valid and widely used, and rosacea patients were involved in their development (2% and 7%, respectively),[57,60] they are theoretically less sensitive than a rosacea-specific HRQoL

Table 1
Commonly used quality-of-life measures evaluating the psychosocial burden of rosacea

Scale	Number of Items	Domains Assessed
Generic QoL measures		
SF-36[61]	36 items	Physical functioning (10 items) Bodily pain (2 items) Emotional wellbeing (5 items) Physical health problems (4 items) Personal or emotional problems (3 items) Social functioning (2 items) Vitality, energy, or fatigue (4 items) General health (5 items)
EQ-5D questionnaire[26]	6 items	Self-care (1 item) Mobility (1 item) Usual activities (1 item) Pain or discomfort (1 item) Anxiety or depression (1 item) plus visual analog scale assessing overall QoL (1 item)
Dermatology-specific QoL measures		
DLQI[60]	10 items	Symptoms and feelings (2 items) Daily activities (2 items) Leisure (2 items) Work and school (1 item) Personal relationships (2 items) Treatment (1 item)
Skindex-29[70]	29 items	Emotions (10 items) Symptoms (7 items) Functioning (12 items)
Rosacea-specific QoL measure		
RosaQoL[23]	21 items	Emotions (11 items) Symptoms (7 items) Functioning (3 items)

Abbreviations: DLQI, Dermatology Life Quality Index; RosaQoL, Rosacea Quality-of-Life Index; SF-36, 36-item Short Form Health Survey.

measure. For example, the DLQI and Skindex-29 include irrelevant factors such as pruritus, which is not a predominant symptom in rosacea. A rosacea-specific HRQoL assessment tool has been developed, but its validity and utility has been questioned.[23,59]

Generic Quality-of-Life Measures

36-item Short Form Health Survey
The 36-item Short Form Health Survey (SF-36) is a validated 36-item QoL instrument centered on 9 concepts: physical functioning, bodily pain, physical health problems, personal or emotional problems, social functioning, vitality, energy or fatigue, general health, and emotional wellbeing.[61] Scored from 0 to 100, higher scores indicate better HRQoL. The SF-36 has been used as an outcome parameter in rosacea clinical trials.[62] In a study with 40 rosacea subjects and 40 controls, the rosacea group had lower QoL in the SF-36 assessed domains of general health perceptions, vitality, emotional sphere, physical functioning, mental health, and bodily pain.[59]

EuroQoL 5-dimension questionnaire
The EQ-5D questionnaire is a validated 2-part QoL instrument. The first part is centered on 5 concepts, including self-care, mobility, usual activities, pain or discomfort, and anxiety or depression.[26] The second part is a 20-cm visual analog scale (VAS) scale scored from 0 to 100, in which respondents are asked to rate their health on a particular day with 100 representing the best possible health and 0 representing the worst possible health. In a metaanalysis using the EQ-5D questionnaire on published and unpublished HRQoL data from Galderma-sponsored studies, of 92 subjects with rosacea, the mean VAS score was 74.0, and the most affected domains were pain or discomfort (31.5% reported moderate to

extreme pain) and anxiety or depression (26.4% reported moderate to extreme anxiety or depression).[22]

Skin-Specific Quality-of-Life Measures

Dermatology Life Quality Index
The DLQI is a validated 10-item QoL instrument that has been used in more than 40 different skin conditions.[60] The DLQI was validated in 120 subjects with dermatologic disease, 2 of whom had rosacea. It is the most commonly used instrument in randomized controlled trials within dermatology.[60] The instrument is centered on 6 domains dealing with symptoms and feelings, daily activities, leisure, work and school, personal relationships, and treatment. Scored from 0 to 30, higher scores indicated greater impact on HRQoL. Although the DLQI has been used in some rosacea studies,[34,63–67] it has only been used twice in randomized head-to-head comparison controlled settings. The first compared doxycycline 40 mg with minocycline 100 mg; the second compared topical 1% ivermectin cream with topical 0.75% metronidazole cream.[68,69]

Skindex-29
The Skindex-29 is a validated 29-item QoL instrument centered on 3 concepts, including emotions, symptoms, and functioning.[70] Scored from 0 to 100, higher scores indicate lower levels of QoL. The Skindex-29 was validated in 685 subjects with dermatologic disease, in which 29 had acne rosacea. Although the Skindex-29 has not been used solely in observational or clinical rosacea trials, in a telephone survey–based study comparing a rosacea-specific QoL measure such as the Rosacea Quality-of-Life Index (RosaQoL) to the Skindex-29, the Skindex-29 was less sensitive than RosaQoL.[71] However, of the 102 subjects called, only 16 completed both QoL instruments. More participants are needed to fully confirm the validity of the results.

Rosacea-Specific Quality-of-Life Measures

Rosacea Quality-of-Life Index
RosaQoL is a validated 21-item QoL instrument centered on 3 hypothesized constructs relating specifically to the psychosocial implications of rosacea symptoms, emotions, and functioning.[23] Each question is scaled from 1 (never) to 5 (all the time) with higher scores signifying greater impairment in HRQoL. RosaQoL was developed from 6 in-depth interviews and later validated in a group of 38 subjects with rosacea. Of the validation group, 92% were white and, based on a subject self-rated severity measure, 24% of subjects

had poor to fair rosacea and 76% had good to excellent rosacea.[23] The instrument had good internal consistency reliability (Cronbach alpha 0.86–0.97) and good reproducibility with an intraclass correlation coefficient ranging from 0.75 to 0.95. However, a key issue with the instrument is its omission of phymatous changes in rosacea, which can be especially debilitating.[72] The development and validation of the RosaQoL was completed in a small population of 38 subjects with narrow demographic, educational, and psychological ranges. It needs to be validated in a broader and more diverse subject population.[23] Also, the finalized score lacks a robust definition of a clinically meaningful difference.[58] Nevertheless, RosaQoL is a popular instrument rivaled only by the DLQI as the HRQoL gold-standard in rosacea studies.[58]

PHARMACOLOGIC INTERVENTIONS AND THEIR IMPACT ON QUALITY OF LIFE

Other than nonpharmacological measures such as the avoidance of potential triggers for flushing, sun protection, and gentle skin care, pharmacologic therapy such as topical agents is the mainstay of rosacea therapy in the United States.[43,73,74] Metronidazole, azelaic acid, oxymetazoline hydrochloride, and brimonidine are the more commonly prescribed first-line agents for rosacea.[43] Other less well-studied topical agents include benzoyl peroxide, erythromycin, clindamycin, sulfacetamide-sulfur, permethrin, and topical retinoids.[43]

In severe cases of rosacea or following the failure of first-line agents, oral antibiotics; low-dose isotretinoin; light-based therapies; and, for ocular rosacea, cyclosporin 0.05% ophthalmic emulsion may be used.[43,75]

There has been no consensus on which standardized tools (eg, HRQoL measurements, participant-assessed improvement in rosacea severity, lesion count, assessment of erythema or telangiectasia) are the best measures of rosacea treatment efficacy.[58] Only a few randomized controlled studies have explored the effect on QoL following pharmacologic treatment (**Table 2**).[63,68,69,76–80] Most studies measuring QoL in rosacea have used skin-specific QoL measures such as the DLQI. Ideally, a rosacea-specific measure such as the RosaQoL should be used, but its validity is still questioned by some opinion leaders.[23,58,59]

Of studies that have used a HRQoL measure as a primary outcome parameter, most have only compared their intervention to placebo. The authors' are aware of only 2 studies that used a

Table 2
Recent randomized controlled trials evaluating the impact of differing antirosacea agents on health-related quality-of-life

Study	Intervention	Study Design	Sample	Sample Size	HRQoL Instrument	Results
Van der Linden et al,[69] 2017	Doxycycline 40 mg vs minocycline 100 mg	Randomized, single-blinded noninferiority trial	Subjects with mild to moderate rosacea	80	RosaQoL	RosaQoL scores decreased for both doxycycline and minocycline by 0.62 and 0.86, respectively (P = .0005)
Bribeche et al,[76] 2015	Topical praziquantel 3% ointment vs placebo	Randomized, prospective, placebo-controlled, single-blind trial	Subjects with mild to moderate rosacea	65	DLQI	Reduction in DLQI from 15.8 to 4.1 in the praziquantel group and from 14.6 to 7.9 in the placebo group (P<.001)
Luger et al,[77] 2015	Topical TDT 068 gel vs placebo	Randomized, prospective, placebo-controlled trial	Erythematotelangiectatic rosacea	61	RosaQoL	Reduction in RosaQoL by 0.08 (SD 0.38) in the TDT 068 gel group and reduction by 0.08 (SD 0.37) in the placebo group (P = .979)
Taieb et al,[68] 2015	Topical ivermectin 1% cream vs topical 0.75% metronidazole cream	Randomized, prospective, active-controlled, investigator-blinded trial	Subjects with moderate to severe papulopustular rosacea	962	DLQI	Reduction in DLQI by 3.92 in the metronidazole group (baseline of 6.05) and reduction by 5.18 in the ivermectin group (baseline of 6.93); no SDs were provided (P<.01)
Stein et al,[80] 2014	Topical ivermectin 1% cream vs placebo	2 randomized, prospective, placebo-controlled, double-blind trials	Subjects with moderate to severe papulopustular rosacea	1371	RosaQoL and DLQI	Ivermectin group: mean change in DLQI was −3.50 (SD 2.77) and −2.30 (SD 2.54) in both trials. Mean change in RosaQoL was 0.64 (SD 0.7) and 0.60 (SD 0.6) in both trials. Placebo group: mean change in DLQI was −2.30 (SD 2.71) and −2.10 (SD 2.48) in both trials. Mean change in RosaQoL was 0.35 (SD 0.5) and 0.35 (SD 0.5) in both trials P<.00001

Chang et al,[78] 2012	Clindamycin phosphate 1.2% and tretinoin 0.025% gel vs placebo	Randomized, prospective, placebo-controlled, double-blind trial	Subjects with papulopustular rosacea with 4 to 50 facial inflammatory lesions	83	RosaQoL	No mean scores of improvements were provided. Only a mean percentage of improved items per questionnaire. The investigators reported no statistically significant difference
Bamford et al,[79] 2012	Zinc sulfate 220 mg vs placebo	Randomized, prospective, placebo-controlled, double-blind, crossover trial	Participants with grade I, II, or III rosacea	25	RosaQoL	Baseline RosaQoL for zinc sulfate group and placebo group was 3.10 and 3.29, respectively. At the end of 3 months, RosaQoL scores reduced to 2.90 and 2.99, respectively, in the zinc sulfate and placebo group(treatment effect estimate was 0.07, $P = .53$)
Weissenbacher et al,[63] 2007	Topical pimecrolimus 1% vs placebo	Randomized, prospective, placebo-controlled, double-blind trial	Subjects with papulopustular rosacea with a rosacea severity score ≥6, an erythema score ≥2, and a scaling score ≥1	40	DLQI	Reduction in DLQI from 5.50 to 3.10 in the pimecrolimus group vs a reduction from 6.70 to 3.70 in the placebo group ($P = .75$)

Abbreviation: SD, standard deviation.

head-to-head comparison in establishing a pharmaceutical intervention's effect on QoL.[68] A total of 962 subjects were randomized to topical 1% ivermectin cream or topical 0.75% metronidazole cream and completed the DLQI at baseline and at the end of the study, week 16. Subjects treated with 1% ivermectin had a higher numerical reduction in their DLQI score than subjects treated with 0.75% metronidazole (−5.18 vs −2.92; P<.01).[68]

ADDRESSING THE PSYCHOSOCIAL IMPACT OF ROSACEA

Rosacea is a condition associated with both physical and psychological comorbidities, which should be considered in the paradigm of a chronic disease, a disease lasting 3 months or more, cannot be prevented by vaccines or cured by medication, nor can it just disappear.[81] Although erythema is commonly reported as its most bothersome symptom, treatment should be tailored to each individual patient and should reflect his or her wishes.[24] Furthermore, antirosacea agents should be accompanied by traditional psychosocial interventions centered on a strong patient-provider relationship. Empathy and open communication is critical in facilitating patient satisfaction.[72] Patient education, reassurance, active self-management, encouraging patients to express their values and desires, and actively helping patients in seeking social support are all often forgotten valuable interventions.[82] In a survey-based study with more than 800 participants with self-reported rosacea, subjects with physician-diagnosed rosacea had more significantly improved symptom control than subjects with un-diagnosed rosacea.[21]

If psychiatric comorbidities are present, the patient should be referred for appropriate counseling and treatment.[83,84] Antidepressants or anxiolytics, and tools such as hypnosis, cognitive-behavioral methods, biofeedback, relaxation training, and meditation have all been noted to help with stress; stress often worsens rosacea's facial flushing.[15,85,86] In a National Rosacea Society survey of more than 700 rosacea subjects, 67% were able to reduce rosacea flares by making a conscious effort to reduce their stress levels. Family and career were the top causes of self-reported emotional stress.[86]

Additional support for patients can be found by connecting with the National Rosacea Society; patients can be directed toward its website (https://www.rosacea.org) for further information. Other worthwhile societies include the Rosacea Support Community[87] with more than 7500 registered members, the American Academy of Dermatology online resources,[88] and the Canadian Skin Patient Alliance.[89] The National Rosacea Society is a nonprofit organization whose mission is to improve the lives of those suffering with rosacea by providing public information, raising awareness of the disease, and encouraging and supporting medical research.[90]

SUMMARY

Rosacea is a chronic disease associated with adverse impact on QoL. The condition is potentially stigmatizing, negatively affects workplace behavior, and is associated with anxiety, depression, and other psychiatric comorbidities. Commonly used QoL measures include rosacea-specific measures such as the RosaQoL and dermatology-specific measures such as the DLQI. Pharmacologic agents, along with social support, empathy, and psychological counseling, aid in decreasing the psychosocial burden of rosacea. Nevertheless, the lack of head-to-head comparisons of interventional efficacy in improving rosacea QoL restricts clinicians' ability to make recommendations based on that outcome. Increasing the awareness of rosacea-related QoL effects is critical in recognizing its status as an impactful chronic disease and in garnering more research interest.

REFERENCES

1. Crawford GH, Pelle MT, James WD. Rosacea: I. Etiology, pathogenesis, and subtype classification. J Am Acad Dermatol 2004;51(3):327–41.
2. McAleer MA, Fitzpatrick P, Powell FC. Papulopustular rosacea: prevalence and relationship to photodamage. J Am Acad Dermatol 2010;63(1):33–9.
3. Berg M. Epidemiological studies of the influence of sunlight on the skin. Photodermatol 1989;6(2):80–4.
4. Elewski BE, Draelos Z, Dréno B, et al. Rosacea - global diversity and optimized outcome: proposed international consensus from the Rosacea International Expert Group. J Eur Acad Dermatol Venereol 2011;25(2):188–200.
5. Tan J, Schöfer H, Araviiskaia E, et al. Prevalence of rosacea in the general population of Germany and Russia - The RISE study. J Eur Acad Dermatol Venereol 2016;30(3):428–34.
6. Lavers I. Rosacea: clinical features and treatment. Nurs Stand 2016;30(31):52–9 [quiz: 60].
7. Tan J, Leyden J, Cribier B, et al. Development and Evaluation of a Rosacea Screening Instrument (Rosascreen). J Cutan Med Surg 2016;20(4):317–22.
8. Little AC, Jones BC, DeBruine LM. Facial attractiveness: evolutionary based research. Philos Trans R Soc Lond B Biol Sci 2011;366(1571):1638–59.

9. Jones BC, Perrett DI, Little AC, et al. Menstrual cycle, pregnancy and oral contraceptive use alter attraction to apparent health in faces. Proc Biol Sci 2005;272(1561):347–54.

10. Jones B, Little A, Penton-Voak I, et al. Facial symmetry and judgements of apparent health. Evol Hum Behav 2001;22(6):417–29.

11. Zebrowitz LA, Montepare JM. Social psychological face perception: why appearance matters. Soc Personal Psychol Compass 2008;2(3):1497.

12. Drummond PD, Quah SH. The effect of expressing anger on cardiovascular reactivity and facial blood flow in Chinese and Caucasians. Psychophysiology 2001;38(2):190–6.

13. Halioua B, Cribier B, Frey M, et al. Feelings of stigmatization in patients with rosacea. J Eur Acad Dermatol Venereol 2017;31(1):163–8.

14. Tan J, Blume-Peytavi U, Ortonne JP, et al. An observational cross-sectional survey of rosacea: clinical associations and progression between subtypes. Br J Dermatol 2013;169(3):555–62.

15. Garnis-Jones S. Psychological aspects of rosacea. J Cutan Med Surg 1998;2(Suppl 4):S4-16-19.

16. Anderson RT, Aaronson NK, Wilkin D. Critical review of the international assessments of health-related quality of life. Qual Life Res 1993;2(6):369–95.

17. Two AM, Wu W, Gallo RL, et al. Rosacea. J Am Acad Dermatol 2015;72(5):749–58.

18. Mikkelsen CS, Holmgren HR, Kjellman P, et al. Rosacea: a clinical review. Dermatol Reports 2016;8(1):6387.

19. National Rosacea Society. Red alert: rosacea awareness month highlights potential increased health risks. Available at: https://www.rosacea.org/press/red-alert-rosacea-awareness-month-highlights-potential-increased-health-risks. Accessed November 24, 2017.

20. Alinia H, Cardwell LA, Moradi Tuchayi S, et al. Symptoms of depression are common in patients with rosacea: PHQ-9 in a diverse rosacea population.

21. Dirschka T, Micali G, Papadopoulos L, et al. Perceptions on the psychological impact of facial erythema associated with rosacea: results of international survey. Dermatol Ther (Heidelb) 2015;5(2):117–27.

22. Bewley A, Fowler J, Schöfer H, et al. Erythema of rosacea impairs health-related quality of life: results of a meta-analysis. Dermatol Ther (Heidelb) 2016;6(2):237–47.

23. Nicholson K, Abramova L, Chren M-M, et al. A pilot quality-of-life instrument for acne rosacea. J Am Acad Dermatol 2007;57(2):213–21.

24. Huynh TT. Burden of disease: the psychosocial impact of rosacea on a patient's quality of life. Am Health Drug Benefits 2013;6(6):348–54.

25. Roosta N, Black DS, Peng D, et al. Skin disease and stigma in emerging adulthood: impact on healthy development. J Cutan Med Surg 2010;14(6):285–90.

26. EuroQol Group. EuroQol–a new facility for the measurement of health-related quality of life. Health Policy 1990;16(3):199–208.

27. Klauder JV. Stigmatization. Arch Dermatol 1938;37(4):650.

28. Ginsburg IH, Link BG. Feelings of stigmatization in patients with psoriasis. J Am Acad Dermatol 1989;20(1):53–63.

29. Major B, O'Brien LT. The social psychology of stigma. Annu Rev Psychol 2005;56(1):393–421.

30. Abram K, Silm H, Maaroos H-I, et al. Risk factors associated with rosacea. J Eur Acad Dermatol Venereol 2010;24(5):565–71.

31. Gupta AK, Chaudhry MM. Rosacea and its management: an overview. J Eur Acad Dermatol Venereol 2005;19(3):273–85.

32. Buechner SA. Rosacea: an update. Dermatology 2005;210(2):100–8.

33. Vardy D, Besser A, Amir M, et al. Experiences of stigmatization play a role in mediating the impact of disease severity on quality of life in psoriasis patients. Br J Dermatol 2002;147(4):736–42.

34. Böhm D, Schwanitz P, Stock Gissendanner S, et al. Symptom severity and psychological sequelae in rosacea: results of a survey. Psychol Health Med 2014;19(5):586–91.

35. Yentzer BA, Fleischer AB. Changes in rosacea comorbidities and treatment utilization over time. J Drugs Dermatol 2010;9(11):1402–6.

36. Gupta MAA, Gupta AKK, Chen SJJ, et al. Comorbidity of rosacea and depression: an analysis of the National Ambulatory Medical Care Survey and National Hospital Ambulatory Care Survey–Outpatient Department data collected by the U.S. National Center for Health Statistics from 1995 to 2002. Br J Dermatol 2005;153(6):1176–81.

37. Hua T-C, Chung P-I, Chen Y-J, et al. Cardiovascular comorbidities in patients with rosacea: a nationwide case-control study from Taiwan. J Am Acad Dermatol 2015;73(2):249–54.

38. Rainer BM, Fischer AH, Luz Felipe da Silva D, et al. Rosacea is associated with chronic systemic diseases in a skin severity dependent manner: results of a case-control study. J Am Acad Dermatol 2015;73(4):604–8.

39. Reich A, Wójcik-Maciejewicz A, Slominski AT. Stress and the skin. G Ital Dermatol Venereol 2010;145(2):213–9.

40. Klaber R, Wittkower E. The pathogenesis of rosacea: a review with special reference to emotional factors. Br J Dermatol 1939;51(12):501–24.

41. Beerman HA. re-evaluation of the rosacea complex. Am J Med Sci 1956;232(4):458–73.

42. Gerber PA, Buhren BA, Steinhoff M, et al. Rosacea: the cytokine and chemokine network. J Investig Dermatol Symp Proc 2011;15(1):40–7.

43. Pelle MT, Crawford GH, James WD. Rosacea: II. Therapy. J Am Acad Dermatol 2004;51(4):499–512.

44. Culp B, Scheinfeld N. Rosacea: a review. P T 2009; 34(1):38–45.

45. Spoendlin J, Bichsel F, Voegel JJ, et al. The association between psychiatric diseases, psychotropic drugs and the risk of incident rosacea. Br J Dermatol 2014;170(4):878–83.

46. Kroenke K, Spitzer RL, Williams JB. The PHQ-9: validity of a brief depression severity measure. J Gen Intern Med 2001;16(9):606–13.

47. Egeberg A, Hansen PR, Gislason GH, et al. Patients with rosacea have increased risk of depression and anxiety disorders: a Danish Nationwide cohort study. Dermatology 2016;232(2):208–13.

48. Dowlati Y, Herrmann N, Swardfager W, et al. A meta-analysis of cytokines in major depression. Biol Psychiatry 2010;67(5):446–57.

49. Miller AH. Depression and immunity: a role for T cells? Brain Behav Immun 2010;24(1):1–8.

50. Maes M. Depression is an inflammatory disease, but cell-mediated immune activation is the key component of depression. Prog Neuropsychopharmacol Biol Psychiatry 2011;35(3):664–75.

51. Sutcigil L, Oktenli C, Musabak U, et al. Pro- and anti-inflammatory cytokine balance in major depression: effect of sertraline therapy. Clin Dev Immunol 2007; 2007:76396.

52. Liu Y, Ho RC, Mak A. The role of interleukin (IL)-17 in anxiety and depression of patients with rheumatoid arthritis. Int J Rheum Dis 2012;15(2):183–7.

53. Kim Y-K, Suh I-B, Kim H, et al. The plasma levels of interleukin-12 in schizophrenia, major depression, and bipolar mania: effects of psychotropic drugs. Mol Psychiatry 2002;7(10):1107–14.

54. Maes M, Song C, Yirmiya R. Targeting IL-1 in depression. Expert Opin Ther Targets 2012;16(11):1097–112.

55. Hopkinson D, Moradi Tuchayi S, Alinia H, et al. Assessment of rosacea severity: a review of evaluation methods used in clinical trials. J Am Acad Dermatol 2015;73(1):138–43.e4.

56. Gessert CE, Bamford JTM. Measuring the severity of rosacea: a review. Int J Dermatol 2003;42(6):444–8.

57. Chren MM, Lasek RJ, Quinn LM, et al. Skindex, a quality-of-life measure for patients with skin disease: reliability, validity, and responsiveness. J Invest Dermatol 1996;107(5):707–13.

58. van Zuuren EJ, Fedorowicz Z, Carter B, et al. Interventions for rosacea. Cochrane Database Syst Rev 2015;(4):CD003262. Available at:. https://doi.org/10.1002/14651858.CD003262.pub5. CD003262. Available at: www.cochranelibrary.com.

59. Tan J, Almeida LMC, Bewley A, et al. Updating the diagnosis, classification and assessment of rosacea: recommendations from the global ROSacea COnsensus (ROSCO) panel. Br J Dermatol 2017;176(2):431–8.

60. Finlay AY, Khan GK. Dermatology Life Quality Index (DLQI)–a simple practical measure for routine clinical use. Clin Exp Dermatol 1994;19(3):210–6.

61. Ware JE, Sherbourne CD. The MOS 36-item short-form health survey (SF-36). I. Conceptual framework and item selection. Med Care 1992;30(6): 473–83.

62. Salamon M, Chodkiewicz J, Sysa-Jedrzejowska A, et al. Quality of life in patients with rosacea. Przegl Lek 2008;65(9):385–9 [in Polish].

63. Weissenbacher S, Merkl J, Hildebrandt B, et al. Pimecrolimus cream 1% for papulopustular rosacea: a randomized vehicle-controlled double-blind trial. Br J Dermatol 2007;156(4):728–32.

64. Shim TN, Abdullah A. The effect of pulsed dye laser on the Dermatology Life Quality Index in erythematotelangiectatic rosacea patients: an assessment. J Clin Aesthet Dermatol 2013;6(4):30–2.

65. Menezes N, Moreira A, Mota G, et al. Quality of life and rosacea: pulsed dye laser impact. J Cosmet Laser Ther 2009;11(3):139–41.

66. Langenbruch AK, Beket E, Augustin M. Quality of health care of rosacea in Germany from the patients perspective: results of the national health care study Rosareal 2009. Dermatology 2011;223(2): 124–30.

67. Aksoy B, Altaykan-Hapa A, Egemen D, et al. The impact of rosacea on quality of life: effects of demographic and clinical characteristics and various treatment modalities. Br J Dermatol 2010;163(4): 719–25.

68. Taieb A, Ortonne JP, Ruzicka T, et al. Superiority of ivermectin 1% cream over metronidazole 0·75% cream in treating inflammatory lesions of rosacea: a randomized, investigator-blinded trial. Br J Dermatol 2015;172(4):1103–10.

69. van der Linden MMD, van Ratingen AR, van Rappard DC, et al. DOMINO, doxycycline 40 mg vs. minocycline 100 mg in the treatment of rosacea: a randomized, single-blinded, noninferiority trial, comparing efficacy and safety. Br J Dermatol 2017;176(6):1465–74.

70. Chren MM, Lasek RJ, Flocke SA, et al. Improved discriminative and evaluative capability of a refined version of Skindex, a quality-of-life instrument for patients with skin diseases. Arch Dermatol 1997; 133(11):1433–40.

71. RosaQoL versus Skindex-29 in measuring quality of life impact in rosacea patients. J Am Acad Dermatol 2005;52(3):P106.

72. Kini SP, Nicholson K, DeLong LK, et al. A pilot study in discrepancies in quality of life among three cutaneous types of rosacea. J Am Acad Dermatol 2010; 62(6):1069–71.

73. Wilkin JK. Use of topical products for maintaining remission in rosacea. Arch Dermatol 1999;135(1): 79–80.

74. Nichols K, Desai N, Lebwohl MG. Effective sunscreen ingredients and cutaneous irritation in patients with rosacea. Cutis 1998;61(6):344–6.

75. Schechter BA, Katz RS, Friedman LS. Efficacy of topical cyclosporine for the treatment of ocular rosacea. Adv Ther 2009;26(6):651–9.

76. Bribeche MR, Fedotov VP, Gladichev VV, et al. Clinical and experimental assessment of the effects of a new topical treatment with praziquantel in the management of rosacea. Int J Dermatol 2015;54(4):481–7.

77. Luger T, Peukert N, Rother M. A multicentre, randomized, placebo-controlled trial establishing the treatment effect of TDT 068, a topical formulation containing drug-free ultra-deformable phospholipid vesicles, on the primary features of erythematotelangiectatic rosacea. J Eur Acad Dermatol Venereol 2015;29(2):283–90.

78. Chang ALS, Alora-Palli M, Lima XT, et al. A randomized, double-blind, placebo-controlled, pilot study to assess the efficacy and safety of clindamycin 1.2% and tretinoin 0.025% combination gel for the treatment of acne rosacea over 12 weeks. J Drugs Dermatol 2012;11(3):333–9.

79. Bamford JTM, Gessert CE, Haller IV, et al. Randomized, double-blind trial of 220 mg zinc sulfate twice daily in the treatment of rosacea. Int J Dermatol 2012;51(4):459–62.

80. Stein L, Kircik L, Fowler J, et al. Efficacy and safety of ivermectin 1% cream in treatment of papulopustular rosacea: results of two randomized, double-blind, vehicle-controlled pivotal studies. J Drugs Dermatol 2014;13(3):316–23.

81. Bernell S, Howard SW. Use your words carefully: what is a chronic disease? Front Public Health 2016;4:159.

82. Bhosle MJ, Kulkarni A, Feldman SR, et al. Quality of life in patients with psoriasis. Health Qual Life Outcomes 2006;4:35.

83. Koo J, Lebwohl A. Psycho dermatology: the mind and skin connection. Am Fam Physician 2001;64(11):1873–8.

84. Azambuja RD. The need of dermatologists, psychiatrists and psychologists joint care in psychodermatology. An Bras Dermatol 2017;92(1):63–71.

85. Shenefelt PD. Psychological interventions in the management of common skin conditions. Psychol Res Behav Manag 2010;3:51–63.

86. Drake L. Stress management can play key role in rosacea control. Newsletter of the National Rosacea Society. Available at: https://www.rosacea.org/rr/2017/winter/stress-management-can-play-key-role-rosacea-control. Accessed November 24, 2017.

87. Pascoe D. Forum page Rosacea Support Community. 2014. 2017. Available at: https://rosacea-support.org/community/index.php?mobile=desktop. Accessed July 11, 2017.

88. Diseases and treatments | American Academy of Dermatology. 2017. https://www.aad.org/public/diseases?redirect. Accessed July 11, 2017.

89. CSPA-Home. 2017. Available at: http://www.canadianskin.ca/en/. Published 2017. Accessed July 11, 2017.

90. National Rosacea Society. About Us | Rosacea.org. 2017. 2017. https://www.rosacea.org/about. Accessed July 6, 2017.

Rosacea Comorbidities

Nora Vera, MD[a], Nupur U. Patel, MS[b], Lucia Seminario-Vidal, MD, PhD[a],*

KEYWORDS

- Rosacea • Comorbidities • Depression • Cardiovascular diseases • Malignancies • Autoimmune
- Neurologic disorders

KEY POINTS

- Several comorbidities have been found to be associated with rosacea, including cardiovascular diseases, depression, gastrointestinal disorders, malignancies, neurologic diseases, and autoimmune conditions.
- Although the exact etiologic factors of rosacea remain to be elucidated, the physiopathology of rosacea is multifactorial, and numerous cell and molecular mechanisms may contribute to the development of rosacea and its comorbidities.
- A chronic inflammatory state may be the underlying mechanism that accounts for its association with cardiovascular diseases.
- Upregulation of matrix metalloproteinases and antimicrobial peptides is the proposed link for rosacea and neurodegenerative disorders.
- Transient receptor potential vanilloid channels are the proposed mediators of neurogenic inflammation that contributes to the physiopathology of rosacea, depression, and migraine.

INTRODUCTION

Rosacea is a common chronic skin disorder characterized by erythema, telangiectasias, flushing, pustules, and fibrosis affecting the central face.[1] Fluctuations in body temperature, psychological factors, ultraviolet exposure, and lifestyle practices, such as alcohol and caffeine intake, are thought to trigger rosacea flares.[1,2] Although the pathogenesis of rosacea is not completely understood, it is regarded as a multifactorial process. Rosacea symptoms are generally thought to be due to an inflammatory process that results from the complex interplay of an aberrant immune system, neurovascular changes, ultraviolet radiation, epidermal barrier dysfunction, and abnormal skin flora.

Rosacea is associated with several comorbidities, including cardiovascular diseases (CVDs), depression, gastrointestinal disorders, malignancies, neurologic conditions, and autoimmune disorders[3–7] (**Fig. 1**). The authors reviewed the literature concerning comorbidities associated with rosacea.

METHODS

A review of English-language articles was performed using PubMed and Google Scholar. Search terms included rosacea, comorbidities, depression, CVD, autoimmune disease, malignancy, and neurologic disorders. Results were categorized by the comorbidity associated with rosacea or by pathophysiologic relationship linking rosacea to a comorbid condition. Results included information since the first description of the association between migraines and rosacea in 1976, as well as more contemporary

Disclosure Statement: Nora Vera, Nupur U. Patel and Lucia Seminario-Vidal have no conflicts to disclose.
[a] Department of Dermatology and Cutaneous Surgery, University of South Florida College of Medicine, 12901 Bruce B. Downs Boulevard, MDC 79, Tampa, FL 33612, USA; [b] Center for Dermatology Research, Department of Dermatology, Wake Forest School of Medicine, Medical Center Boulevard, Winston-Salem, NC 27157-1071, USA
* Corresponding author.
E-mail address: luciasem@health.usf.edu

Dermatol Clin 36 (2018) 115–122
https://doi.org/10.1016/j.det.2017.11.006

derm.theclinics.com

The Burden of Rosacea

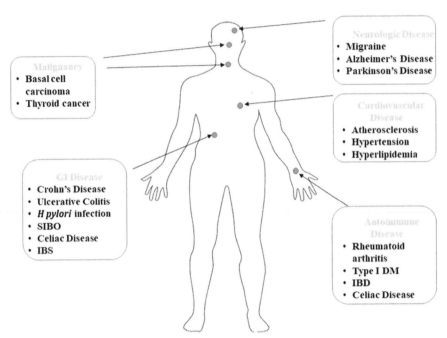

Fig. 1. An overview of comorbidities most commonly seen with rosacea. *H. pylori*, *Helicobacter pylori*.

epidemiologic data, etiologic data, and retrospective reviews conducted over the past 30 years.

ROSACEA-ASSOCIATED COMORBIDITIES
Cardiovascular Diseases

Inflammation plays a key role in the pathogenesis of rosacea and is an established risk factor in the development of atherosclerosis and its complications. Rosacea and atherosclerosis share the upregulation of cathelicidin in inflammatory cells and low serum paraoxonase-1 (PON-1) activity.[1,8–10] In the skin and vasculature, apart from its antimicrobial activity, cathelicidin functions as an immune modulator, inducing expression of inflammatory genes, leading to cytokine and chemokine liberation from local cells and leukocytes.[8] Injection of mice with cathelicidin peptide fragments from the skin of patients with rosacea produced a rosacea-like dermatitis.[11] Furthermore, cathelicidin-deficient mice were protected against atherosclerosis.[12]

PON-1 is an antioxidant enzyme that protects against atherosclerosis by metabolizing lipid peroxides and preventing the oxidative modification of serum lipoproteins. PON-1–knockout mice developed atherosclerosis faster than their wild-type litter mates on a high-fat diet.[13] In subjects

with CVD, PON-1 activity is decreased by half compared with healthy subjects.[14,15] Serum PON-1 enzyme activity was lower in subjects with rosacea than in healthy controls.[10] Altogether, these studies suggest that an increase in cathelicidin and oxidative stress are contributing factors to the pathogenesis of rosacea and atherosclerosis. However, only a few studies have investigated whether patients with rosacea have higher risk of CVD.[7,16–18] One study noted increased prevalence of hyperlipidemia, hypertension, metabolic syndrome, and CVD in patients with rosacea.[17] A retrospective review of National Health Insurance Research Database in Taiwan revealed that patients with rosacea were more likely to have dyslipidemia (odds ratio [OR] 1.41, 95% CI 1.36–1.46), coronary artery disease (OR 1.35, 95% CI 1.29–1.41), and hypertension (OR 1.17, 95% CI 1.12–1.21) compared with controls.[7] Although these studies indicated a higher prevalence of CVD and CVD risk factors in patients with rosacea, the increased frequency of hypercholesterolemia in that patient population may have been confounded by higher incidence of alcohol consumption and smoking.[16] More recently, a Danish population-based study determined that rosacea was not independently associated with CV risk.[18] Future studies are needed to elucidate the relationship between CVD and rosacea.

Oncologic Disorders

Studies linking malignancies and rosacea are scarce.[6,19–22] In a study assessing the association between personal history of rosacea and risk of incident cancers, there was a significant association between personal history of rosacea and thyroid cancer. In terms of skin cancer, rosacea was associated with an elevated risk of basal cell carcinoma (**Fig. 2**).[6] The investigators suggested that underlying inflammation may be a potential link explaining these associations.

In a Danish study assessing cancer incidence in rosacea patients compared with the general population, rosacea patients had increased incidence of nonmelanoma skin cancer (NMSC), breast cancer, and hepatic cancer.[22] In an older study assessing the incidence of skin cancers in patients with rosacea, patients with rosacea were not more likely to have skin cancer or solar degeneration compared with control subjects.[21] However, in more recent studies, personal history of rosacea was associated with an increased risk of NMSC.[6,22] The increased risk of NMSC should be carefully interpreted in these studies because many of these subjects also had a history of

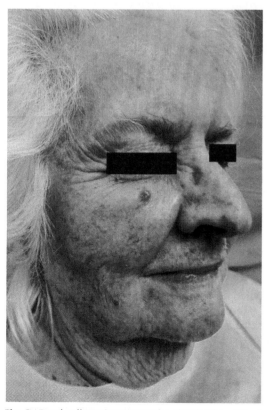

Fig. 2. Basal cell carcinoma on the cheek of a patient with rosacea.

extensive exposure to ultraviolet radiation.[23] A potential explanation for the link between NMSC and rosacea may be that the skin barrier dysfunction in rosacea patients results in reduced endogenous trans-urocanic acid, leading to an increase in ultraviolet radiation–induced DNA damage and phototumorigenesis.[24]

Neurologic and Mental Disorders

Neurologic and mental disorders are prevalent in patients with rosacea; the underlying mechanisms remain unknown.[3,25–31] Neurovascular dysregulation and neurogenic inflammation may play a role in the pathophysiology of rosacea, migraine, depression, and anxiety.[32] Transient receptor potential ion channels of vanilloid (TRPV) type are mediators of neurogenic inflammation. They are implicated in peripheral pain perception and are expressed in keratinocytes, endothelial cells, and sensory neurons in the brain. TRPVs are nonselective cation channels activated by heat, ethanol, spicy foods, and other chemicals.

Peripheral inflammation in the gut of rats induces anxiety-like and depression-like behaviors, which are mediated by activation of TRPV-1.[33] Furthermore, inhibition of TRPV-1 has an antidepressant effect.[34,35] TRPV-1 channels are increased in the trigeminal fibers of chronic migraine patients and in the skin of erythematotelangiectatic and phymatous rosacea patients.[36,37] TRPV-1 receptor activation leads to a release of calcitonin gene-related peptide from trigeminal terminals during severe migraine attacks, leading to vasodilatation and neurogenic pain.[38,39] Gene expression of calcitonin gene-related peptide is significantly increased in erythematotelangiectatic rosacea compared with telangiectatic photoaging and controls.[40] These studies suggest that TRPV-1 may play a role in the pathogenesis of rosacea and the neurologic and mental health comorbidities associated with rosacea. Whether activation of TRPV-1 in rosacea-prone skin induces depression in humans remains to be investigated. TRPV1 may represent a new molecular target for treatment of these associated conditions.

Depression

Rosacea has been associated with higher depression scores, feelings of low self-esteem, stigmatization, and decreased quality of life.[3,25,26,41] Treatment of rosacea results in improved quality of life.[26] In a metaanalysis assessing Dermatology Life Quality Index (DLQI) in rosacea, subjects with severe rosacea had worse mean DLQI scores than subjects with moderate rosacea.[25] A nationwide survey of adult patients with rosacea that evaluated the willingness to pay (WTP) amount for a complete cure, revealed that the average sum was approximately $3770.[42] WTP is a method that reflects an individual's burden of disease. In this study, WTP was higher in female patients and patients with severe disease. Both WTP and DLQI scores were lower in patients with rosacea compared with patients with vitiligo. Compared with other dermatologic disorders, the impact of rosacea on health-related quality of life was comparable to acne and psoriasis.[43]

Migraines

The first description of the association between rosacea and migraines dates from 1976 when it was found that 44% of patients with rosacea suffered from migraines compared with 13% of controls.[44] Subsequent studies have since revealed similar associations.[28,29] Larger and more contemporary work has demonstrated an overall association between rosacea and migraine in women (adjusted OR 1.22, 95% CI 1.16–1.29) but not in men. This association was most pronounced in patients with severe migraines, 50 years of age or older.[30] A nationwide cohort study from Denmark reported the prevalence of migraines among patients with rosacea as 12.1%, and demonstrated an increased risk of new onset migraine in patients with rosacea compared with the general population. This risk was the highest in patients with ocular rosacea, reaching 69% (adjusted hazard ratio [HR] 1.69, 95% CI 1.43–1.99).[27]

Neurodegenerative diseases

Inflammation, increased matrix metalloproteinases activity, and antimicrobial peptides are involved in the pathogenesis of neurodegenerative disorders, including Alzheimer disease and Parkinson disease (PD). These factors are also implicated in the pathogenesis of rosacea. One study noted that rosacea patients had an increased risk of dementia, particularly Alzheimer disease, compared with subjects who did not have the skin condition.[45] Another study reported a 2-fold increased risk of PD in the rosacea population compared with the general population. Patients who received tetracyclines to treat rosacea had a decreased risk of PD, regardless of the presence of rosacea at time of PD diagnosis.[31]

Gastrointestinal Disease

Small intestinal bacterial overgrowth (SIBO), *Helicobacter pylori*, and irritable bowel disease (IBD) have been described to occur in conjunction with rosacea; however, findings are inconsistent between studies.[4] Resident gut bacteria may play a role in this co-occurrence, potentially serving as the underlying trigger to an exaggerated immune response. Improvements in IBD and rosacea symptoms with oral metronidazole support this notion. Rosacea symptoms may also be mediated by inflammatory factors in the digestive tract. Bradykinin, implicated as the plasma kallikrein–kinin system (PKKS), is activated in patients with intestinal inflammation. Activation of PKKS is also increased in rosacea patients.[46]

Small intestinal bacterial overgrowth

There is increased prevalence of rosacea in patients with SIBO. Rosacea may be triggered by SIBO due to increased circulating cytokines, particularly tumor necrosis factor-alpha.[47,48] In 1 study, 46% of rosacea subjects were diagnosed with SIBO; treatment with rifaximin resulted in complete resolution of cutaneous symptoms in 78% of the cohort.[47] Similar results have been achieved in small studies, though whether improvement in symptoms was the result of SIBO eradication or decreased systemic immune stimulation is unclear.[47–49] It is hypothesized that remission may have been achieved with rifaximin due to its direct antimicrobial effects on gut bacteria, rather than systemic absorption or antiinflammatory activity.[50]

Irritable bowel disease

Evidence suggests that an aberrant innate immune response to certain stimuli leads to gastrointestinal neurogenic inflammation and, consequently, the manifestations of IBD. Similarly, robust immune activation triggered by various stimuli is thought to underlie the neurogenic inflammation and vascular dysregulation that manifests in rosacea symptoms.[48] Concurrent inflammatory skin diseases, such as psoriasis, can contribute to the clinical picture of IBD; thus, if rosacea is regarded as an inflammatory cutaneous condition, its relationship to IBD is plausible.[51]

Multiple reports have described the co-occurrence of IBD and rosacea. A large observational case-control analysis suggested that patients with IBD are at a 3-fold increased risk of developing rosacea. This observed risk correlated with IBD severity, suggesting that the observed association between rosacea and IBD is outcome-specific, as opposed to a general inflammatory or autoimmune disease.[52] Results of large-scale population studies confirm this association. In a nationwide cohort study of the Danish population, rosacea was associated with an increased prevalence of IBD and increased risk of new-onset IBD. Similarly, results of a nationwide cohort study based out of Taiwan found a significant association between rosacea and IBD. The cumulative incidences of IBD were compared between patients with and without rosacea. The incidence of IBD was higher in the rosacea group than in the cohort without rosacea. Rosacea and male gender were independently associated with IBD. The incidence rates of IBD decreased with the increased use of antibiotics in subjects with rosacea; however, this finding was not deemed statistically significant.[53] The association between rosacea and IBD is further supported by the genetic overlap between rosacea and IBD on the histocompatibility complex class II protein-coding gene HLADRB1*03:01.[4]

Helicobacter pylori infection

As with SIBO, the role of H pylori in the pathogenesis of rosacea remains controversial. Though studies report an increased prevalence of H pylori in rosacea subjects, others have failed to demonstrate this association. The effect of H pylori eradication on rosacea symptoms is variable, with recent metaanalysis failing to reveal significant association between rosacea and H pylori.[54] In this metaanalysis, studies using urea breath test for the diagnosis of H pylori infection yielded a stronger association between the 2 conditions compared with studies using serologic tests.[54] Interpretation of observed rosacea improvement with treatment of H pylori is complicated because both conditions can be treated with oral antibiotics. Disagreement in findings may be explained by differing strains of H pylori and contributions to pathogenesis by specific virulence factors, such as cytotoxin-associated gene A.[55]

Irritable bowel syndrome

New data have linked irritable bowel syndrome (IBS) and rosacea for the first time. A nationwide cohort study noted increased risk of new-onset IBS in subjects with rosacea. Adjusted HR revealed significant associations between rosacea and IBS (HR 1.34, 95% CI 1.19 – 1.50).[4] Though these findings may be a result of misdiagnosed IBS, they may also reflect yet another comorbidity of rosacea.

Autoimmune Diseases

Recent genome-wide association studies have identified shared risk loci between rosacea and autoimmune diseases such as type 1 diabetes mellitus (T1DM), rheumatoid arthritis (RA), and celiac disease.[56] Three HLA alleles are associated with rosacea (**Table 1**). The DRB1*03:01-DQB1*02:01-DQA1*05:01 haplotype has been associated with T1DM and HLA-DQB1*02:01 has previously been associated with celiac disease.[56] These findings were further confirmed in a population-based study. After adjustment for

Table 1
Statistically significant P-values of 3 alleles associated with rosacea in discovery and replication groups

HLA Allele	P-Value	
	Discovery group (n = 22,952)	Replication group (n = 29,48)
HLA-DRB1*03:01	$P = 1.0 \times 10^{(-8)}$	$P = 4.4 \times 10^{(-6)}$
HLA-DQB1*02:01	$P = 1.3 \times 10^{(-8)}$	$P = 7.2 \times 10^{(-6)}$
HLA-DQA1*05:01	$P = 1.4 \times 10^{(-8)}$	$P = 7.6 \times 10^{(-6)}$

Data from Chang ALS, Raber I, Xu J, et al. Assessment of the genetic basis of rosacea by genome-wide association study. J Invest Dermatol 2015;135:1548–55.

smoking and socioeconomic status, subjects with rosacea had significantly increased ORs for T1DM, celiac disease, multiple sclerosis, and RA. These associations were observed in women and only reached statistical significance for RA in men.[5] This study may highlight shared etiopathogenesis of genetic origin.

SUMMARY

A growing body of literature exists that links rosacea to multiple comorbidities. However, the strength and interpretation of these associations remains to be clearly delineated. Existing literature seems to implicate the potential for underlying pathogenic mechanisms responsible for multiple disease states. Neural dysregulation, aberrant immune activation, systemic inflammation, in addition to genetic and environmental factors, are all potential contributors to a seemingly multifactorial disease. A paradigm of the natural history of rosacea and its comorbidities is illustrated in **Fig. 3**.

The inconsistency of relationships between rosacea and comorbidities within the literature may be limited by the statistical power of the studies and use of self-reported data, as well as the observational and retrospective nature of the analyses. However, large-scale epidemiologic studies have revealed significant associations with plausible shared mechanisms, implying there is a need for further exploration of these comorbidities. Many of the larger-scale studies are based in Denmark, which consists of a largely white population, therefore limiting the generalizability of the data to other ethnic groups and associated skin types.

The potential for rosacea as a prognostic indicator for certain disease states should be explored.

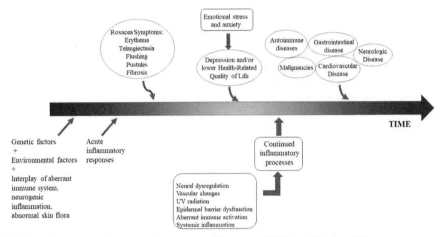

Fig. 3. Paradigm of the natural history of rosacea and its comorbidities. UV, ultraviolet.

The potential for control of comorbid conditions to ameliorate rosacea symptoms or vice versa may be a direction for future research. Additionally, the question of whether physical examination findings of rosacea symptoms could predict treatment responses or mandate further screening tests for comorbidities remains to be explored.

REFERENCES

1. Steinhoff M, Schauber J, Leyden JJ. New insights into rosacea pathophysiology: a review of recent findings. J Am Acad Dermatol 2013;69:15–26.
2. Del Rosso JQ, Gallo RL, Kircik L, et al. Why is rosacea considered to be an inflammatory disorder? The primary role, clinical relevance, and therapeutic correlations of abnormal innate immune response in rosacea-prone skin. J Drugs Dermatol 2012;11: 694–700.
3. Gupta MA, Gupta AK, Chen SJ, et al. Comorbidity of rosacea and depression: an analysis of the National Ambulatory Medical Care Survey and National Hospital Ambulatory Care Survey–Outpatient Department data collected by the U.S. National Center for Health Statistics from 1995 to 2002. Br J Dermatol 2005;153:1176–81.
4. Egeberg A, Weinstock LB, Thyssen EP, et al. Rosacea and gastrointestinal disorders: a population-based cohort study. Br J Dermatol 2017;176:100–6.
5. Egeberg A, Hansen PR, Gislason GH, et al. Clustering of autoimmune diseases in patients with rosacea. J Am Acad Dermatol 2016;74:667–72.e2.
6. Li W-Q, Zhang M, Danby FW, et al. Personal history of rosacea and risk of incident cancer among women in the US. Br J Cancer 2015;113:520–3.
7. Hua TC, Chung PI, Chen YJ, et al. Cardiovascular comorbidities in patients with rosacea: a nationwide case-control study from Taiwan. J Am Acad Dermatol 2015;73:249–54.
8. Edfeldt K, Agerberth B, Rottenberg ME, et al. Involvement of the antimicrobial peptide LL-37 in human atherosclerosis. Arterioscler Thromb Vasc Biol 2006;26:1551–7.
9. Durrington PN, Mackness B, Mackness MI. Paraoxonase and atherosclerosis. Arterioscler Thromb Vasc Biol 2001;21:473–80.
10. Takci Z, Bilgili SG, Karadag AS, et al. Decreased serum paraoxonase and arylesterase activities in patients with rosacea. J Eur Acad Dermatol Venereol 2015;29:367–70.
11. Yamasaki K, Di Nardo A, Bardan A, et al. Increased serine protease activity and cathelicidin promotes skin inflammation in rosacea. Nat Med 2007;13: 975–80.
12. Döring Y, Drechsler M, Wantha S, et al. Lack of neutrophil-derived CRAMP reduces atherosclerosis in mice. Circ Res 2012;110:1052–6.
13. Shih DM, Gu L, Xia YR, et al. Mice lacking serum paraoxonase are susceptible to organophosphate toxicity and atherosclerosis. Nature 1998;394:284–7.
14. Ayub A, Mackness MI, Arrol S, et al. Serum paraoxonase after myocardial infarction. Arterioscler Thromb Vasc Biol 1999;19:330–5.
15. Mackness MI, Harty D, Bhatnagar D, et al. Serum paraoxonase activity in familial hypercholesterolaemia and insulin-dependent diabetes mellitus. Atherosclerosis 1991;86:193–9.
16. Duman N, Ersoy Evans S, Atakan N. Rosacea and cardiovascular risk factors: a case control study. J Eur Acad Dermatol Venereol 2014;28:1165–9.
17. Rainer BM, Fischer AH, Luz Felipe da Silva D, et al. Rosacea is associated with chronic systemic diseases in a skin severity-dependent manner: results of a case-control study. A portion of this work was presented at the Society for Investigative Dermatology Annual Meeting in Albuquerque, New Mexico, May 7-10. J Am Acad Dermatol 2015;73:604–8.

18. Egeberg A, Hansen PR, Gislason GH, et al. Assessment of the risk of cardiovascular disease in patients with rosacea. J Am Acad Dermatol 2016;75:336–9.

19. Margolin L. Severe rosacea associated with colon cancer recurrence. Int J Dermatol 2004;43:213–4.

20. Friedman GD, Oestreicher N, Chan J, et al. Antibiotics and risk of breast cancer: up to 9 years of follow-up of 2.1 million women. Cancer Epidemiol Biomarkers Prev 2006;15:2102–6.

21. Dupont C. Rosacea is not associated with skin cancer. Arch Dermatol 1986;122:1099.

22. Egeberg A, Fowler JF, Gislason GH, et al. Rosacea and risk of cancer in Denmark. Cancer Epidemiol 2017;47:76–80.

23. Aldrich N, Gerstenblith M, Fu P, et al. Genetic vs environmental factors that correlate with rosacea. JAMA Dermatol 2015;151:1213.

24. Barresi C, Stremnitzer C, Mlitz V, et al. Increased sensitivity of histidinemic mice to UVB radiation suggests a crucial role of endogenous urocanic acid in photoprotection. J Invest Dermatol 2011;131:188–94.

25. Bewley A, Fowler J, Schöfer H, et al. Erythema of rosacea impairs health-related quality of life: results of a meta-analysis. Dermatol Ther (Heidelb) 2016;6:237–47.

26. Moustafa F, Lewallen RS, Feldman SR. The psychological impact of rosacea and the influence of current management options. J Am Acad Dermatol 2014;71:973–80.

27. Egeberg A, Ashina M, Gaist D, et al. Prevalence and risk of migraine in patients with rosacea: a population-based cohort study. J Am Acad Dermatol 2017;76:454–8.

28. Ramelet AA. Rosacea: a reaction pattern associated with ocular lesions and migraine? Arch Dermatol 1994;130:1448.

29. Berg M, Lidén S. Postmenopausal female rosacea patients are more disposed to react with migraine. Dermatology 1996;193:73–4.

30. Spoendlin J, Voegel JJ, Jick SS, et al. Migraine, triptans, and the risk of developing rosacea: a population-based study within the United Kingdom. J Am Acad Dermatol 2013;69:399–406.

31. Egeberg A, Hansen PR, Gislason GH, et al. Exploring the association between rosacea and Parkinson disease. JAMA Neurol 2016;73:529.

32. Brennan K, Charles A. An update on the blood vessel in migraine. Curr Opin Neurol 2010;23:266–74.

33. Chen J, Winston JH, Fu Y, et al. Genesis of anxiety, depression, and ongoing abdominal discomfort in ulcerative colitis-like colon inflammation. Am J Physiol Regul Integr Comp Physiol 2015;308:R18–27.

34. Manna SSS, Umathe SN. A possible participation of transient receptor potential vanilloid type 1 channels in the antidepressant effect of fluoxetine. Eur J Pharmacol 2012;685:81–90.

35. Socala K, Wla P. Evaluation of the antidepressant- and anxiolytic-like activity of α-spinasterol, a plant derivative with TRPV1 antagonistic effects, in mice. Behav Brain Res 2016;303:19–25.

36. Del Fiacco M, Quartu M, Boi M, et al. TRPV1, CGRP and SP in scalp arteries of patients suffering from chronic migraine. J Neurol Neurosurg Psychiatry 2015;86:393–7.

37. Sulk M, Seeliger S, Aubert J, et al. Distribution and expression of non-neuronal transient receptor potential (TRPV) ion channels in rosacea. J Invest Dermatol 2012;132:1253–62.

38. Meng J, Ovsepian SV, Wang J, et al. Activation of TRPV1 mediates calcitonin gene-related peptide release, which excites trigeminal sensory neurons and is attenuated by a retargeted botulinum toxin with anti-nociceptive potential. J Neurosci 2009;29:4981–92.

39. Goadsby PJ, Edvinsson L. The trigeminovascular system and migraine: studies characterizing cerebrovascular and neuropeptide changes seen in humans and cats. Ann Neurol 1993;33:48–56.

40. Helfrich YR, Maier LE, Cui Y, et al. Clinical, histologic, and molecular analysis of differences between erythematotelangiectatic rosacea and telangiectatic photoaging. JAMA Dermatol 2015;151:825.

41. Halioua B, Cribier B, Frey M, et al. Feelings of stigmatization in patients with rosacea. J Eur Acad Dermatol Venereol 2017;31:163–8.

42. Beikert FC, Langenbruch AK, Radtke MA, et al. Willingness to pay and quality of life in patients with rosacea. J Eur Acad Dermatol Venereol 2013;27:734–8.

43. Cresce ND, Davis SA, Huang WW, et al. The quality of life impact of acne and rosacea compared to other major medical conditions. J Drugs Dermatol 2014;13:692–7.

44. Tan SG, Cunliffe WJ. Rosacea and migraine. Br Med J 1976;1:21.

45. Egeberg A, Hansen PR, Gislason GH, et al. Patients with rosacea have increased risk of dementia. Ann Neurol 2016;79:921–8.

46. Kendall SN. Remission of rosacea induced by reduction of gut transit time. Clin Exp Dermatol 2004;29:297–9.

47. Parodi A, Paolino S, Greco A, et al. Small intestinal bacterial overgrowth in rosacea: clinical effectiveness of its eradication. Clin Gastroenterol Hepatol 2008;6:759–64.

48. Weinstock LB, Steinhoff M. Rosacea and small intestinal bacterial overgrowth: prevalence and response to rifaximin. J Am Acad Dermatol 2013;68:875–6.

49. Weinstock LB. Rosacea in Crohn's disease: effect of rifaximin. J Clin Gastroenterol 2011;45:295–6.

50. Drago F, De Col E, Agnoletti AF, et al. The role of small intestinal bacterial overgrowth in rosacea: a 3-year follow-up. J Am Acad Dermatol 2016;75(3): e113–5.

51. Kim M, Choi KH, Hwang SW, et al. Inflammatory bowel disease is associated with an increased risk of inflammatory skin diseases: a population-based cross-sectional study. J Am Acad Dermatol 2017; 76:40–8.

52. Spoendlin J, Karatas G, Furlano RI, et al. Rosacea in patients with ulcerative colitis and Crohn's disease: a population-based case-control study. Inflamm Bowel Dis 2016;22(3):680–7.

53. Wu C-Y, Chang Y-T, Juan C-K, et al. Risk of inflammatory bowel disease in patients with rosacea: results from a nationwide cohort study in Taiwan. J Am Acad Dermatol 2017;76:911–7.

54. Jørgensen A-HR, Egeberg A, Gideonsson R, et al. Rosacea is associated with Helicobacter pylori: a systematic review and meta-analysis. J Eur Acad Dermatol Venereol 2017 [Epub ahead of print]. Available at: http://doi.wiley.com/10.1111/jdv.14352. Accessed September 4, 2017.

55. Argenziano G, Donnarumma G, Iovene MR, et al. Incidence of anti-Helicobacter pylori and anti-CagA antibodies in rosacea patients. Int J Dermatol 2003;42:601–4.

56. Chang ALS, Raber I, Xu J, et al. Assessment of the genetic basis of rosacea by genome-wide association study. J Invest Dermatol 2015;135:1548–55.

Rosacea Triggers
Alcohol and Smoking

Hossein Alinia, MD[a], Sara Moradi Tuchayi, MD, MPH[a], Nupur U. Patel, MS[a],
Nishit Patel, MD[b], Olabola Awosika, MD, MS[c], Naeim Bahrami, PhD[a,d],
Leah A. Cardwell, MD[a,*], Irma Richardson, MHA[a], Karen E. Huang, MS[a],
Steven R. Feldman, MD, PhD[a,e,f]

KEYWORDS

• Rosacea • Triggers • Alcohol • Smoking • Tobacco • Cigarettes • Nicotine

KEY POINTS

- Clear associations have not been made in literature between the cutaneous inflammatory disorder rosacea and triggers such as alcohol, smoking, and sun exposure.
- Increased severity of disease was significantly associated with number of cigarettes smoked in previous smokers and marginally associated with patients who consumed 6 or more alcoholic beverages in 1 day.
- Subjects who experienced increased sun exposure due to their employment had significantly increased disease severity.
- Although the relationship between these triggers and rosacea remains to be elucidated, these results may contribute to the development of practical recommendations for trigger avoidance in rosacea patients.

INTRODUCTION

Although multiple factors contribute to the pathophysiology of rosacea, it is considered a dynamic inflammatory process that begins with recurrent dilatation of cutaneous vessels and later neovascularization, causing erythema and telangiectasias of the face.[1–4] A variety of triggers are thought to induce or exacerbate rosacea. These triggers include alcohol, spicy food, hot beverages, tobacco, acetones, high temperatures, sun exposure, and stress.[5,6] A limited number of studies have evaluated the prevalence of smoking in rosacea and the specific influence smoking may have on disease symptoms.[4,7,8] Although alcohol is a trigger of the transient flushing that often accompanies rosacea, the association between alcohol intake and rosacea development and severity remains unclear.[6,9–12] Sun exposure is thought to be a trigger for rosacea, but the relationship between rosacea severity and sun exposure needs to be better elucidated.[6,11] In one large-scale patient self-reported survey study, sun exposure was the most common

Disclosure: See last page of article.
[a] Center for Dermatology Research, Department of Dermatology, Wake Forest School of Medicine, Medical Center Boulevard, Winston-Salem, NC 27157-1071, USA; [b] Department of Dermatology and Cutaneous Surgery, University of South Florida College of Medicine, University of South Florida, 12901 Bruce B. Downs Boulevard, MDC 79, Tampa, FL 33612, USA; [c] Department of Dermatology, The George Washington Medical Faculty Associates, 2150 Pennsylvania Avenue Northwest, 2B-427, Washington, DC 20037, USA; [d] Department of Biomedical Engineering, Virginia Polytechnic Institute and State University, Wake Forest University, Medical Center Boulevard, Winston Salem, NC 27157-1071, USA; [e] Department of Pathology, Wake Forest School of Medicine, Medical Center Boulevard, Winston-Salem, NC 27157-1071, USA; [f] Department of Public Health Sciences, Wake Forest School of Medicine, Medical Center Boulevard, Winston-Salem, NC 27157-1071, USA
* Corresponding author.
E-mail address: lcardwell06@gmail.com

Dermatol Clin 36 (2018) 123–126
https://doi.org/10.1016/j.det.2017.11.007

trigger identified.[13] However, other reports in the literature do not support this finding.[6] Likewise, although some patients report that season changes are a trigger for rosacea, the relationship between specific seasons and severity of rosacea is unclear.[13] The authors aim to better characterize associations between rosacea severity and triggers, such as smoking, alcohol consumption, sun exposure, and season changes.

METHODS

Subjects were adult patients at the Wake Forest Baptist Medical Center dermatology clinic from 2011 to 2014 who received a clinical diagnosis of rosacea (*International Classification of Diseases, Ninth Revision* [ICD-9] code: 695.3) from a Wake Forest dermatologist. Institutional Review Board approval was obtained before initiation of this study. Data were collected from October 2014 until February 2015. Eligible rosacea patients were identified using Wake Forest Baptist Hospital's Transitional Data Warehouse and the electronic medical record. Children were excluded because rosacea is not typically present in children, and the measures used were not validated in children.

In order to recruit subjects to complete the survey in person, 165 patients were contacted via phone. A total of 46 subjects who came to the office to validate the self-assessment tool were recruited to complete the survey during the same visit. A presurvey letter was mailed to 432 subjects to inform them that they would receive the survey via mail. Twenty subjects declined to receive the survey. Surveys were mailed to 412 subjects. Sixteen surveys were returned by the post office because of address changes. A total of 195 surveys (149 via mail and 46 in person) were completed and analyzed. Participants completed quality-of-life assessments, a demographics questionnaire, and a survey that included questions about alcohol and tobacco use, seasonal allergies, and daily sun exposure. All participants who completed the survey by mail also completed a previously validated self-assessment tool. Patients selected images to identify the severity of their symptoms; categories included erythema, papulopustular lesions, ocular symptoms, and nasal involvement. Scores ranged from 2 (least severe) to 8 (most severe). Results were reported using descriptive statistics. Regression analysis was performed to identify independent outcome predictors.

RESULTS
Smoking

One hundred eighty-two subjects responded to the smoking survey questions, and 47% of subjects had smoked at least 100 cigarettes in their lives. In patients who were previous smokers, there was a significant relationship between the severity of disease and number of cigarettes smoked ($P = .037$, F ratio = 4.51, n = 73). There was no significant relationship between the years since quitting and severity of disease ($P = .38$, F ratio = 0.77, n = 75). Forty-seven percent of subject responders had smoked at least 100 cigarettes in their lifetime but were not current smokers. There was no significant relationship between the severity of disease and having smoked greater than or less than 100 cigarettes in their lives ($P = .24$, t ratio = -1.16, df = 180). Ninety percent (n = 101) of subjects who responded to current smoking status were not current smokers. Among patients who were actively smoking, the mean age at start of smoking was 17.37 years with SD of 2.69 years. There was no linear association between the severity of disease and the age at which smoking began ($P = .79$, F ratio = 0.08, n = 82). The authors used the current age as covariate for this analysis. There was no association between having smoked 30 days before survey completion and the severity of disease ($P = .60$, F ratio = 0.26, n = 90).

Alcohol

One hundred seventy-eight subjects responded to alcohol-related survey questions. One hundred thirty-nine had consumed alcoholic beverages in the past year. Among those who consumed alcohol, there was no relationship between number of drinks 30 days before completing the survey and disease severity ($P = .91$, F ratio = 0.01, n = 133). There was no association between the number of drinks consumed per day and disease severity ($P = .91$, F ratio = 0.01, n = 128). There were marginally significant relationships between consumption of 6 or more drinks and presence of severe disease ($P = .06$, t ratio = 1.51).

Other Triggers

Subjects with a sun-based job requirement had more severe rosacea compared to those who did not have a sun-based job ($P = .04$, t ratio = -1.70). Of the 167 subjects who answered questions regarding seasonal impact, 52% (n = 87) were unsure of a specific season triggering their rosacea. Of the remaining 80 patients, 3% reported that their rosacea was more severe in spring; 50% reported greater severity in the summer; 3% reported greater severity in the fall; and 46% reported greater severity in the winter.

DISCUSSION

We investigated multiple triggers for rosacea patients using self-reported demographic and social history data. In this study, nearly half of study subjects (47%) had smoked at least 100 cigarettes in their life but were not current smokers; there was no significant relationship between the number of cigarettes smoked and severity of disease. Prior studies have published similar results; for instance, one study noted that rosacea was predominantly a disease of nonsmokers; however, this study did not perform separate analysis of ex-smokers and nonsmokers.[14] According to another study, ex-smokers for more than 1 year were more frequently affected by rosacea than active smokers.[4,7] A retrospective cohort study noted an increased risk of rosacea associated with past smoking compared with never smoking, and a decreased risk associated with current smoking. Increasing pack-years of smoking was associated with elevated risk of rosacea among past smokers ($P = .003$) and decreased risk of rosacea among current smokers ($P<.0001$).[15] In contrast, another study noted higher prevalence of smoking among rosacea patients and higher prevalence of erythematotelangiectatic rosacea among active smokers, citing that this relationship between smoking and rosacea might be due to the angiogenic effects of nicotine.[4] Given the incongruity of these studies, the effect of smoking on inflammatory skin diseases such as rosacea remains unclear.

Most subjects who responded to the alcohol survey questions had consumed alcoholic beverages within the past year. Those who had consumed 6 or more drinks in one or more days had increased disease severity compared with those who did not. Previous reports demonstrate that alcohol may accelerate the progression of rosacea.[9] However, although alcohol is a well-documented trigger for flushing in rosacea, the association between alcohol consumption and rosacea development and severity remains controversial. In an American survey study, less than 2% of subjects who were being treated for alcoholism had rosacea. In a French survey study, only 5.6% of subjects had rosacea, and 35% attributed rosacea flares to alcohol consumption.[9,12]

In our study, 40 out of the 80 subjects who reported worse rosacea depending on the season noted that their disease worsened in the summer. Because sunlight is thought to be a trigger of rosacea, this finding may be due to the increased sun exposure during the summer months. The association between sun exposure and rosacea is also corroborated by increased severity of disease reported in patients who have outdoor jobs with extensive sun exposure. These findings are supported by data from the National Rosacea Society, in which 71% of more than 700 rosacea patients said their condition was affected by changes in seasons, summer being the most common, and 57% of respondents reported that their symptoms were worse during the summer.[16]

There are several limitations to the study. The study population consisted of university dermatology clinic patients who may not be representative of patients in the general population. However, the authors' hospital system does not require referrals and cares for a large percentage of the surrounding community. Although only 44.1% of patients responded to the survey, nonresponders matched responders for age and sex. The findings may inform physician counseling practices, because patients may be provided with practical measures for managing their rosacea, such as decreasing heavy alcohol consumption over short periods of time and increasing sun protection, especially in the summer months. Although results may vary, many patients may benefit from these practical measures, and rosacea patient outcomes may improve over time.

DISCLOSURE STATEMENT

S.R. Feldman is a speaker for Janssen and Taro. He is a consultant and speaker for Galderma, Stiefel/GlaxoSmithKline, Abbott Labs, Leo Pharma Inc. S.R. Feldman has received grants from Galderma, Janssen, Abbott Labs, Amgen, Stiefel/GlaxoSmithKline, Celgene, and Anacor. He is a consultant for Amgen, Baxter, Caremark, Gerson Lehrman Group, Guidepoint Global, Hanall Pharmaceutical Co Ltd, Kikaku, Lilly, Merck & Co Inc, Merz Pharmaceuticals, Mylan, Novartis Pharmaceuticals, Pfizer Inc, Qurient, Suncare Research, and Xenoport. He is on an advisory board for Pfizer Inc. S.R. Feldman is the founder and holds stock in Causa Research and holds stock and is majority owner in Medical Quality Enhancement Corporation. He receives Royalties from UpToDate and Xlibris. H. Alinia, S.M. Tuchayi, N.U. Patel, N. Patel, O. Awosika, N. Bahrami, L.A. Cardwell, I. Richardson, and K.E. Huang have no conflicts of interest to disclose.

REFERENCES

1. Crawford GH, Pelle MT, James WD. Rosacea: I. Etiology, pathogenesis, and subtype classification. J Am Acad Dermatol 2004;51:327–41 [quiz: 342–4]. Available at: http://linkinghub.elsevier.com/retrieve/pii/S0190962204008448. Accessed September 4, 2017.

2. Wilkin J, Dahl M, Detmar M, et al. Standard classification of rosacea: report of the National Rosacea Society Expert Committee on the classification and staging of rosacea. J Am Acad Dermatol 2002;46:584-7. Available at: http://www.ncbi.nlm.nih.gov/pubmed/11907512. Accessed September 4, 2017.

3. Del Rosso JQ. Advances in understanding and managing rosacea: part 2: the central role, evaluation, and medical management of diffuse and persistent facial erythema of rosacea. J Clin Aesthet Dermatol 2012;5:26-36.

4. Kucukunal A, Altunay I, Arici JE, et al. Is the effect of smoking on rosacea still somewhat of a mystery? Cutan Ocul Toxicol 2016;35(2):110-4.

5. Culp B, Scheinfeld N. Rosacea: a review. P T 2009;34:38-45.

6. Abram K, Silm H, Maaroos H-I, et al. Risk factors associated with rosacea. J Eur Acad Dermatol Venereol 2010;24:565-71.

7. Breton AL, Truchetet F, Véran Y, et al. Prevalence analysis of smoking in rosacea. J Eur Acad Dermatol Venereol 2011;25:1112-3.

8. Smith JB, Smith SB. Cigarette smoking and inflammatory skin disease. The good and the bad. Arch Dermatol 1997;133:901-2.

9. Higgins E, du Vivier A. Alcohol intake and other skin disorders. Clin Dermatol 1999;17:437-41.

10. Higgins EM, du Vivier AW. Alcohol abuse and treatment resistance in skin disease. J Am Acad Dermatol 1994;30:1048.

11. Jaworek AK, Wojas-Pelc A, Pastuszczak M. Aggravating factors of rosacea. Przegl Lek 2008;65:180-3 [in Polish].

12. Rosset M, Oki G. Skin diseases in alcoholics. Q J Stud Alcohol 1971;32:1017-24.

13. Rosacea Triggers Survey. Available at: https://www.rosacea.org/patients/materials/triggersgraph.php. Accessed November 28, 2017.

14. Mills CM, Marks R. Environmental factors influencing rosacea. Clin Exp Dermatol 1996;21:172-3. Available at: http://www.ncbi.nlm.nih.gov/pubmed/8759214. Accessed September 4, 2017.

15. Li S, Cho E, Drucker AM, et al. Cigarette smoking and risk of incident rosacea in women. Am J Epidemiol 2017;186:38-45.

16. Drake L. Survey reports sun season hardest on rosacea symptoms. Available at: https://www.rosacea.org/rr/1996/spring/article_3.php. Accessed November 28, 2017.

Evaluating and Optimizing the Diagnosis of Erythematotelangiectatic Rosacea

Mohammed D. Saleem, MD, MPH*, Jonathan K. Wilkin, MD

KEYWORDS

- Diagnostic • History • Physical • Differential

KEY POINTS

- An accurate diagnosis and classification are fundamentally essential for clear communication among researchers and health care providers.
- Early recognition improves clinical outcomes and quality of life and reduces morbidity.
- A thorough history and physical examination are critical in distinguishing between rosacea and other diagnoses that may present similarly.

INTRODUCTION

Rosacea is a common chronic inflammatory dermatosis with a prevalence between 0.1% and 10%.[1–4] It is associated with a high incidence of embarrassment, social anxiety, depression, and decreased quality of life.[5] Despite psychosocial complications, rosacea is often undiagnosed, misdiagnosed, undertreated, or mistreated, especially in skin of color.[2,6–14]

Rosacea is defined by recognizable morphologic features; no histologic or diagnostic tests are available.[15–17] The National Rosacea Society (NRS) consensus is the most widely used rosacea criteria (**Table 1**).[18] In this paradigm, optimal evaluation and diagnosis of rosacea incorporate current scientific knowledge (increase diagnostic sensitivity) and exclude diseases with similar phenotypic features (increase diagnostic specificity).[19]

An accurate diagnosis and classification are fundamentally essential for clear communication among researchers and health care providers.[20] In addition, early recognition improves clinical outcomes, improves quality of life, and reduces morbidity.[5,21–25] The purpose of this article is to describe an optimal clinical approach to diagnosing the most prevalent rosacea subtype, erythematotelangiectatic rosacea (ETR), which commonly occurs with ocular rosacea, but much less frequently occurs with the other rosacea subtypes.[3,26–28] The article begins by summarizing the current diagnostic foundation set by NRS and adds diagnostic specificity by incorporating a critical question, "what is not rosacea?" The authors briefly highlight shared features of ETR and papulopustular rosacea (PPR).

ROSACEA: CURRENT CLINICAL FOUNDATION

Rosacea is a diagnostic term that describes a chronic heterogeneous group of signs and symptoms primarily affecting the convexities of the midface.[29] Persistent erythema lasting at least 3 months with a tendency to spare periocular skin is the most important primary feature of ETR and PPR; flushing, papules, pustules, and

Disclosure: See last page of article.
University of Florida College of Medicine, PO Box 100277, Gainesville, FL 32610-0277, USA
* Corresponding author.
E-mail address: msaleem@g.clemson.edu

Dermatol Clin 36 (2018) 127–134
https://doi.org/10.1016/j.det.2017.11.008

derm.theclinics.com

Table 1
Rosacea diagnostic and classification criteria

Diagnostic Criteria: Requires the Presence of ≥1 Primary Feature in a Centrofacial Distribution	
Primary Features	Secondary Features
Transient erythema	Ocular manifestations
Nontransient erythema	Burning or stinging
Telangiectases	Phymatous changes
Papules and pustules	Dry appearance, plaques, edema, or peripheral location
Classification Criteria	
Subtype	Characteristics
Erythematotelangiectatic	Flushing and persistent central facial erythema with or without telangiectasia
Papulopustular	Persistent or transient central facial papules and/or pustules often in same stage of development
Phymatous	Thickening skin, irregular surface nodularities and enlargement, usually beginning as patulous follicles; may occur on the nose, chin, forehead, cheeks, or ears
Ocular	Foreign body sensation in the eye, burning or stinging, dryness, itching, ocular photosensitivity, blurred vision, telangiectasia of the sclera or other parts of the eye, or periorbital edema

telangiectasias are additional features.[16] Pediatric rosacea presents similarly, except sebaceous gland hyperplasia does not occur.[30,31] The mean age of onset, in children, is 6 years of age with an average delay in diagnosis of 3 years.[32] Rosacea is rarely diagnosed adequately in skin of color, partially because facial erythema and telangiectasias are less visually apparent.[9,10,33]

Flushing is often the first sign, typically limited to the convexities of the midface, especially the cheeks.[34–36] Extrafacial flushing occurs in 24% of subjects, often involving the throat or superior chest.[1,35] Flushing can be idiopathic or may be triggered by external factors; this manifestation may also be accompanied by heat (97%), skin tension (36%), sweating (30%), burning/stinging (25%), and/or pruritus.[1,16,35] Environmental, dietary, and topical factors may predispose and exacerbate erythema and skin sensitivity manifesting as pruritus, stinging, burning, or xerosis.[37–40]

Erythematotelangiectatic Rosacea

ETR is characterized by persistent centrofacial erythema, transient erythema (flushing), and sensitive skin with or without telangiectasias.[16,30,41,42] Flushing, in response to internal or external stimuli, is often a prominent and bothersome feature.[16] Flushing may become more frequent and longer in duration as the disease progresses.[43] The skin of subjects with ETR typically appears dry and rough with possible fine scale; these findings

occur more frequently in ETR than in other rosacea subtypes.[35] Although treatments have been developed for the redness of ETR, intolerance due to skin irritation of topicals often limits adherence.[44] Nasal involvement may serve as a marker for predicting progression to more severe rosacea.[45]

Papulopustular Rosacea

PPR is characterized by the presence of small domed inflammatory papules and pustules often on a background of persistent centrofacial erythema with universal periocular sparing.[41,44] Two-thirds of patients with PPR in one series had a preceding diagnosis of ETR.[35] Flushing and skin sensitivity are common, suggesting that PPR commonly coexists with ETR.[16] Papules and pustules tend to be located on the cheeks (80%), nose (67%), chin (47%), forehead (40%), and neck (7%).[35] The papules are persistent in 58% of patients, whereas the remaining 42% have transient papules and pustules that occur with flares.[35] Transient papules associated with flares often have substantial resolution of the palpable component within 2 weeks; residual erythema is much slower to fade.[35] Similar to acne, inflammatory lesions may occasionally rupture, resulting in extension of erythema. Rarely, PPR with ETR may have repeated episodes of inflammation and tissue remodeling that can lead to chronic lymphedema.[46,47] Despite treatment, the risk of relapse is 40% after cessation of treatment, often requiring maintenance therapy.[48–50]

CLINICAL EVALUATION
General

A primary feature of centrofacial distribution establishes the diagnosis of rosacea with high sensitivity.[24] Diagnostic specificity can be increased with a thorough history and physical examination, with special attention to primary features. Up to 40% may have a family history of rosacea.[51] Medications, occupation, and cumulative sun exposure are important in differentiating rosacea from drug-induced and extrinsic photoaging (UV-induced skin changes). Complete review of systems is critical in ruling out systemic conditions.

Secondary features are frequently present and supportive of rosacea diagnosis. Ocular rosacea frequently (50%) coexists with cutaneous rosacea, especially with ETR; a third of patients with ocular rosacea develop potential sight-threatening complications.[13,14] Foreign body sensation, gritty sensation, pruritus, tearing, or inability to wear contact lenses are frequent manifestations of ocular rosacea. Skin sensitivity presents with mild pruritus and topical intolerance. When erythema is patchy and severe pruritus is the primary complaint, patch testing is warranted and can be diagnostic when allergy to topicals is suspected.[16] Edema can accompany episodic exacerbation; rarely, solid facial edema (persistent, nonpitting edema) is a complication of PPR. Ocular rosacea occurs more frequently in patients with intense or frequent flushing. A patient with ETR should be queried regarding symptoms of ocular rosacea.

Flushing (Transient Erythema)

Flushing or transient erythema is defined as sensation of warmth accompanied by erythematous change in skin due to vascular smooth muscle relaxation. Neural-mediated flushing is often accompanied by sweating and palpitations, in contrast to "dry flush," in which a vasoactive agent, endogenous or exogenous, acts directly on smooth muscle without any effect on the sweat glands. Dry flush may be caused by doxorubicin, cisplatin, interferon alfa, metoclopramide, and ethanol. Wet flushing can be caused by vasodilators, such as calcium channel blockers, nitrites, vancomycin, cyclosporine, tamoxifen, and nonsteroidal anti-inflammatory drugs.[52] Patients with rosacea have more flushing with use of vasodilators such as niacin or methyl nicotinate compared with patients with other dermatologic conditions with similar clinical appearance.[53] Emotional flushing in response to an appropriate stimulus, such as social embarrassment, is normal and transient. In the United States, the prevalence of "hot or climacteric flushes" in women aged 40 to 65 was 88%, and exacerbating factors were similar to triggers of rosacea.[1,35,54] In the absence of other primary features, isolated flushing is not a reason to label a patient with prerosacea because most cases never go on to develop rosacea.[44] Severe prolonged flushing followed with pallor and diaphoresis, or accompanied by diarrhea, wheezing, headache, palpitation, and/or dizziness should prompt consideration for a neoplastic process such as pheochromocytoma or carcinoid syndrome (**Table 2**).[36,53,55–59] In the absence of

Table 2
Carcinoid syndrome characteristics

Carcinoid Syndrome Characteristics	
Age	Often >60 y of age
Flushing distribution	Face, neck, and trunk
Triggers	Alcohol, emotional stress, and certain foods
Associated symptoms with flushing	Diarrhea (42%), diarrhea plus dyspnea or wheezing (38%), generalized severe pruritus (8%), other[a]
Late complications	Pellagra (20%), scleroderma (8%), PPR (13%), rhinophyma (2%)[b]

When neuroendocrine tumors metastasize, metabolic products can bypass the liver and manifest with cutaneous findings. The earliest manifestation is flushing, occurring in 95% of cases. Tumors arising embryologically from the foregut produce pink to red flushing; in contrast, midgut tumors produce cyanotic flushing. Associated diarrhea, dyspnea, or wheezing differentiates it from other causes of flushing. Chronic repeated episodes of flushing are associated with the development of fixed erythema, telangiectasia, and connective tissue hypertrophy such as that seen with carcinoid syndrome or rosacea. Consequently, carcinoid syndrome is often initially misdiagnosed as rosacea.

[a] Carcinoid syndrome can also present with hives that are very pruritic, accompanied by hypotension and tachycardia during episodes.

[b] Carcinoid tumor metabolizes significant tryptophan to produce serotonin. Consequently, a relative deficiency in tryptophan can result manifesting as skin fragility, erythema, and hyperpigmentation over knuckles and shins.

Data from Refs.[36,55–57,59]

Table 3
Red flags associated with flushing that require further diagnostic consideration

Red Flags	Diagnostic Consideration	Laboratory Marker
Unintentional weight loss	Neuroendocrine tumor	See below
Wheezing	Carcinoid syndrome	Urine 5-HIAA
Diarrhea	Carcinoid syndrome	Urine 5-HIAA
	VIPoma	Serum VIP
	Mastocytosis[a]	Serum tryptase or urine n-methylhistamine
Severe hypertension, tachycardia, and/or sense of impending doom	Pheochromocytoma[b]	Urine catecholamines
Hematuria, flank pain	Renal cell carcinoma	Kidney ultrasound
Generalized pruritus after shower or history of unusual clots (Budd-Chiari syndrome, renal vein thrombosis, and so on)	Polycythema vera	Erythrocytosis

Abbreviations: 5-HIAA, 5-hydroxyindoleacetic acid; VIP, vasoactive intestinal peptide.
[a] Consider when flushing coincides with hypotension and urticarial pigmentosa. In the pediatric population, urticarial pigmentosa eruption occurs in 90% of children with mastocytosis.
[b] Hypertension can be sustained or paroxysmal.

concerning features, the diagnosis of ETR is often straightforward and does not require extensive workup (**Table 3**).

Nontransient Erythema and Telangiectasia

Extrinsic photoaging
A close examination is necessary to differentiate between fine telangiectasia and simple erythema. In dark skin, erythema can be difficult to appreciate; inquiring specifically about transient episodes of erythema and skin sensitivity is critical in such populations. Retroauricular skin, a site expected to be devoid of UV exposure and rosacea, can be used to assess baseline skin redness; in contrast, the sternocleidomastoid area can be assessed for erythema secondary to additive

Table 4
Comparison of features associated with erythematotelangiectatic rosacea and UV-induced changes

	Erythematotelangiectatic Rosacea	Extrinsic Photoaging[a]
Shared features	Facial pigmentation, telangiectasias, skin roughness and dryness, facial erythema that spares periocular skin	
Distribution of erythema	Predominantly central (79%)	Photo-exposed skin (57%) (preauricular and mandibular region)
Extrafacial involvement	Rare	Upper chest
Transient erythema[b]	88%	35% (similar to control group)
Nontransient erythema	92%	65%
Associations	Flushing, burning, stinging	Photodamage, skin cancer

Recently, ETR was clinically, histologically, and molecularly compared with skin associated with extrinsic skin aging. Subjects with erythema associated with extrinsic photoaging were less likely to experience flushing, burning, or stinging.
[a] The investigators used the term telangiectatic photoaging to denote extrinsic photoaging. The authors use the term extrinsic photoaging to provide consistency with other studies. The study was a case-control study involving 46 cases and 11 controls. Inclusion criteria required patients undergo facial biopsy; subjects with a history of skin cancer or previous biopsy are more likely to enroll than younger subjects or women. All subjects recruited were older men. Because of selection bias, the demographics and prevalence of skin cancer are not representative of the true population.
[b] Subjects with moderate or severe flushing were excluded. No conclusions should be drawn between differences in the occurrence of flushing in either population.
Data from Helfrich YR, Maier LE, Cui Y, et al. Clinical, histologic, and molecular analysis of differences between erythematotelangiectatic rosacea and telangiectatic photoaging. JAMA Dermatol 2015;151(8):825.

sum of both extrinsic photoaging and baseline skin redness. The malar region can then be examined to determine what potential additional contribution to the erythema beyond the sum of baseline skin redness and photoaging can be attributed to rosacea (**Table 4**).[60,61] Centrofacial telangiectasias are characteristic of extrinsic skin aging independent of ethnicity.[62–66] The relationship between ETR and photoaging has consistently been reported, and the clinical distinction can be subtle.[20,35,60,64,67,68] Features suggestive of photoaging include fine wrinkles, skin roughness and dryness, irregular pigmentation, telangiectasia, sallowness, and lentigines.[69]

Other considerations

Atopic and seborrheic dermatitis are frequent causes of facial erythema. Seborrheic dermatitis presents with macular erythema and greasy scales involving the scalp, eyebrows, or retroauricular region.[70] Atopic dermatitis is characterized by pruritic papules and plaques, xerosis, keratosis pilaris, and hyperlinearity of the plantar and palmar surfaces.[70] Facial erythema, often involving the malar or seborrheic regions, is common in dermatomyositis and lupus erythematosus (LE) and may precede systemic symptoms by years. In LE, like in rosacea, cutaneous features may be exacerbated by sun exposure. Acute localized LE, precipitated by sun exposure, may manifest as well-defined malar erythema with sparing of the nasolabial folds and periocular region. Nasolabial sparing and persistent erythema for weeks help differentiate LE from seborrheic dermatitis and photosensitive dermatitis, respectively.[71,72] Well-demarcated malar erythema is also common in dermatomyositis. However, in dermatomyositis, the erythema is of a violaceous or dusky hue and frequently involves the periorbital region.[51,73,74]

SUMMARY

Multiple conditions have similar clinical features as ETR. A thorough history and physical examination can provide important clues to narrow the diagnosis. Early recognition and adequate treatment may improve clinical outcomes and patient satisfaction.

DISCLOSURE

Dr. M.D. Saleem has nothing to disclose. Dr. J.K. Wilkin has been a consultant or consultant and board member for the following companies: Aclaris, Adocia SA, Aisling Capital LLC, Aldeyra Therapeutic Allergan Sales, LLC, Almirall SA, Amicus Therapeutics, Amryt Pharmaceuticals, Anacor Pharmaceuticals, Aponia Laboratories, Inc., Applied Biology, Inc., Arcutis, Inc., Braintree Laboratories, Inc., Brickell Biotech, CanFite, CapGenesis LLC, Capstone Development Services, Cara Therapeutics, Inc., Cassiopea S.p.A., Castle Creek Pharmaceuticals, LLC, Chugai Pharma USA, Inc., CinRx Pharma, Clarus Ventures, LLC, Chromaderm Inc., Clementia Pharmaceuticals Inc., CODA Therapeutics, Inc., Corcept Therapeutics, Inc., Cowen and Company, Crescita Therapeutics Inc., Dalhousie University, Deb Group LTD, Demira Inc., Dermex Pharmaceutical Inc., Dermtreat ApS, DFB Soria, LLC, Dipexium Pharmaceuticals, Dr. Reddy's Laboratories SA Swiss, Dr. Reddy's Laboratories LTD (India), DUSA Pharmaceuticals Effexus Pharmaceutical, LLC, Ervin Epstein, Extera Partners, Foamix, Galderma Research & Development FR, Genentech, Inc., Genogen, Inc., GlaxoSmithKline LLC, Genfit, Halozyme, Inc., Hildred Capital Partners LLC, istogen Inc., Human Matrix Sciences, LLC, Incyte Corporation, Immune Pharmaceuticals, Innovimmune Biotherapuetics Holding LLC, Insmed Incorporated, Kythera Biopharmaceuticals, LEO Pharma, LEIO Corporation, Lehigh Valley Technologies, Inc., Lilly USA LLC, Linkverse SRI, Lithera Inc., Livionex Inc., Louis Simo S.A.S., MC2 Biotek, McLean Hunt Consulting Group, Macrocure Ltd, Mayne Pharma Group, Medimetriks Pharmaceuticals, MedImmune/AstraZeneca, MediWound Ltd, Meiji Seika Pharma Co. LTD, MitsubishiTanabe Pharma, Mylan Pharmaceuticals In., NDA Partners LLC, NanoBio Corporation, Neokera, LLC, NextScience LLC, Nobelpharma, NovaLead Pharma Pvt Ltd, Novan, Inc., Nuvo Research, Inc., Orenova, Orphaderm LTD, Otsuka Pharmaceutical Co., Palvella Therapeutics LLC, Patagonia Pharmaceuticals LLC, Patara Pharma LLC, PellaPharm, Inc., Pfizer Inc., Photocure ASA, Pierre Fabre Dermatologie, Promius Pharma LLC, Prugen Inc., Quark Pharmaceuticals, Inc., Quellthera Inc., Realm Therapeutics., Raglan Acquisitions LTD, Revance Therapeutics, Roviant Sciences, Inc., Scioderm Inc., Sebacia, Inc., Seton Pharmaceuticals, Sienna Biopharmaceuticals, Inc., Slayback Pharma, Smith & Nephew, Sol-Gel Technologies, Squarex LLC, Stiefel Laboratories, Inc., Sun Pharma Advanced Research Co. LTD, Sun Pharma Global FZE, Symbiomix Therapeutics, LLC, Taro Pharmaceuticals, Teva Branded Pharmaceutical Products, The Medicines Company, Therapeutics, Inc., Thesan Pharmaceuticals, Tigercat Pharma, Inc., Tolmar, Inc., Trevi Therapeutics, Inc., True NorthTherapeutics, Two B Pharmaceuticals, Ulthera, Inc., Valeant Pharmaceuticals North America, Velius LLC, Verrica Pharmaceuticals Inc., Viamet Pharmaceuticals, Inc., ViDAC Pharma, Ltd.,

Vyome Biosciences Pvt. LTD, Water Street Health-care Partners, Watson Pharmaceuticals, Xenon Pharmaceuticals Inc., XenoPort, Inc., XOMA Ziarco Pharma Ltd, Zurex Pharma, Inc. He has been a member of the board of the National Rosacea Society which originated in contracted Public Awareness Efforts of rosacea and Metrogel and evolved into the current 501(c)(3) nonprofit organization generously supported by Galderma among other corporate donors.

REFERENCES

1. Tan J, Berg M. Rosacea: current state of epidemiology. J Am Acad Dermatol 2013;69(6 suppl 1):S27–35.
2. Kligman AM. An experimental critique on the state of knowledge of rosacea. J Cosmet Dermatol 2006;5(1):77–80.
3. Kyriakis KP, Palamaras I, Terzoudi S, et al. Epidemiologic aspects of rosacea. J Am Acad Dermatol 2005;53(5):918–9.
4. McAleer MA, Fitzpatrick P, Powell FC. Papulopustular rosacea: prevalence and relationship to photodamage. J Am Acad Dermatol 2010;63(1):33–9.
5. Moustafa F, Lewallen RS, Feldman SR. The psychological impact of rosacea and the influence of current management options. J Am Acad Dermatol 2014;71(5):973–80.
6. Quarterman MJ, Johnson DW, Abele DC, et al. Ocular rosacea. Signs, symptoms, and tear studies before and after treatment with doxycycline. Arch Dermatol 1997;133(1):49–54.
7. Ghanem VC, Mehra N, Wong S, et al. The prevalence of ocular signs in acne rosacea: comparing patients from ophthalmology and dermatology clinics. Cornea 2003;22(3):230–3. Available at: http://www.ncbi.nlm.nih.gov/pubmed/12658088. Accessed January 16, 2017.
8. Browning DJ, Rosenwasser G, Lugo M. Ocular rosacea in blacks. Am J Ophthalmol 1986;101(4):441–4.
9. Rosen T, Stone MS. Acne rosacea in blacks. J Am Acad Dermatol 1987;17(1):70–3.
10. Alexis AF. Rosacea in patients with skin of color: uncommon but not rare. Cutis 2010;86(2):60–2. Available at: http://www.ncbi.nlm.nih.gov/pubmed/20919596. Accessed January 15, 2017.
11. Tidman MJ. Improving the management of rosacea in primary care. Practitioner 2014;258(1775):27–30, 3. Available at: http://www.ncbi.nlm.nih.gov/pubmed/25591285. Accessed January 15, 2017.
12. Tanzi EL, Weinberg JM. The ocular manifestations of rosacea. Cutis 2001;68(2):112–4. Available at: http://www.ncbi.nlm.nih.gov/pubmed/11534911. Accessed January 15, 2017.
13. Vieira ACC, Höfling-Lima AL, Mannis MJ. Ocular rosacea–a review. Arq Bras Oftalmol 2012;75(5):363–9. Available at: http://www.ncbi.nlm.nih.gov/pubmed/23471336. Accessed January 15, 2017.
14. Vieira AC, Mannis MJ. Ocular rosacea: common and commonly missed. J Am Acad Dermatol 2013;69(6 suppl 1):S36–41.
15. Fonseca GP, Brenner FM, Muller Cde S, et al. Nailfold capillaroscopy as a diagnostic and prognostic method in rosacea. An Bras Dermatol 2011;86(1):87–90. Available at: http://www.ncbi.nlm.nih.gov/pubmed/21437527. Accessed January 16, 2017.
16. Crawford GH, Pelle MT, James WD. Rosacea: I. Etiology, pathogenesis, and subtype classification. J Am Acad Dermatol 2004;51(3):327–41.
17. Powell FC. The histopathology of rosacea: "where's the beef?'. Dermatology 2004;209(3):173–4.
18. Wilkin J, Dahl M, Detmar M, et al. Standard classification of rosacea: report of the National Rosacea Society expert committee on the classification and staging of rosacea. J Am Acad Dermatol 2002;46(4):584–7.
19. Tan J, Steinhoff M, Berg M, et al. Shortcomings in rosacea diagnosis and classification. Br J Dermatol 2017;176(1):197–9.
20. Odom R. Rosacea, acne rosacea, and actinic telangiectasia: in reply [16]. J Am Acad Dermatol 2005;53(6):1103–4.
21. Jaworek AK, Wojas-Pelc A, Pastuszczak M. [Aggravating factors of rosacea]. Przegl Lek 2008;65(4):180–3 [in Polish] Available at: http://www.ncbi.nlm.nih.gov/pubmed/18724544. Accessed January 15, 2017.
22. Elewski BE, Draelos Z, Dréno B, et al. Rosacea—global diversity and optimized outcome: proposed international consensus from the Rosacea International Expert Group. J Eur Acad Dermatol Venereol 2011;25(2):188–200.
23. Mackley CL, Thiboutot DM. Diagnosing and managing the patient with rosacea. Cutis 2005;75(4 Suppl):25–9. Available at: http://www.ncbi.nlm.nih.gov/pubmed/15916227. Accessed January 16, 2017.
24. Wilkin J, Dahl M, Detmar M, et al. Standard grading system for rosacea: report of the National Rosacea Society expert committee on the classification and staging of rosacea. J Am Acad Dermatol 2004;50(6):907–12.
25. McDonnell JK, Tomecki KJ. Rosacea: an update. Cleve Clin J Med 2000;67(8):587–90. Available at: http://www.ncbi.nlm.nih.gov/pubmed/10946455. Accessed January 16, 2017.
26. Abram K, Silm H, Oona M. Prevalence of rosacea in an Estonian working population using a standard classification. Acta Derm Venereol 2010;90(3):269–73.
27. Khaled A, Hammami H, Zeglaoui F, et al. Rosacea: 244 Tunisian cases. Tunis Med 2010;88(8):597–601.

Available at: http://www.ncbi.nlm.nih.gov/pubmed/20711968. Accessed January 15, 2017.

28. Berg M, Lidén S. An epidemiological study of rosacea. Acta Derm Venereol 1989;69(5):419–23. Available at: http://www.ncbi.nlm.nih.gov/pubmed/2572109. Accessed February 24, 2017.

29. Powell FC, Raghallaigh SN. Dermatology. In: Bolognia JL, Jorizzo JL, Schaffer JV, editors. Rosacea and related disorders. 3rd edition. London: Saunders; 2012. p. 561–9.

30. Kroshinsky D, Glick SA. Pediatric rosacea. Dermatol Ther 2006;19(4):196–201.

31. Lacz NL, Schwartz RA. Rosacea in the pediatric population. Cutis 2004;74(2):99–103. Available at: http://www.ncbi.nlm.nih.gov/pubmed/15379362. Accessed January 15, 2017.

32. Donaldson KE, Karp CL, Dunbar MT. Evaluation and treatment of children with ocular rosacea. Cornea 2007;26(1):42–6.

33. Al-Dabagh A, Davis SA, McMichael AJ, et al. Rosacea in skin of color: not a rare diagnosis. Dermatol Online J 2014;20(10). Available at: http://www.ncbi.nlm.nih.gov/pubmed/25526008.

34. Marks R, Jones EW. Disseminated rosacea. Br J Dermatol 1969;81(1):16–28. Available at: http://www.ncbi.nlm.nih.gov/pubmed/4236713. Accessed January 16, 2017.

35. Tan J, Blume-Peytavi U, Ortonne JP, et al. An observational cross-sectional survey of rosacea: clinical associations and progression between subtypes. Br J Dermatol 2013;169(3):555–62.

36. Wilkin JK. Oral thermal-induced flushing in erythematotelangiectatic rosacea. J Invest Dermatol 1981;76(1):15–8. Available at: http://www.ncbi.nlm.nih.gov/pubmed/6450809. Accessed January 16, 2017.

37. Lonne-Rahm SB, Fischer T, Berg M. Stinging and rosacea. Acta Derm Venereol 1999;79(6):460–1. Available at: http://www.ncbi.nlm.nih.gov/pubmed/10598761. Accessed January 16, 2017.

38. Draelos ZD. Facial hygiene and comprehensive management of rosacea. Cutis 2004;73(3):183–7. Available at: http://www.ncbi.nlm.nih.gov/pubmed/15074346. Accessed January 15, 2017.

39. Jappe U, Schnuch A, Uter W. Rosacea and contact allergy to cosmetics and topical medicaments—retrospective analysis of multicentre surveillance data 1995-2002. Contact Dermatitis 2005;52(2):96–101.

40. Guzman-Sanchez DA, Ishiuji Y, Patel T, et al. Enhanced skin blood flow and sensitivity to noxious heat stimuli in papulopustular rosacea. J Am Acad Dermatol 2007;57(5):800–5.

41. Gauwerky K, Klövekorn W, Korting HC, et al. Rosacea. J Dtsch Dermatol Ges 2009;7(11):996–1003.

42. Metzler-Wilson K, Toma K, Sammons DL, et al. Augmented supraorbital skin sympathetic nerve activity responses to symptom trigger events in rosacea patients. J Neurophysiol 2015;114(3):1530–7.

43. National Rosacea Society. Living with rosacea. Dermatol Nurs 2007;19(3):274–5. Available at: http://www.ncbi.nlm.nih.gov/pubmed/17626507. Accessed January 15, 2017.

44. Powell FC. Clinical practice. Rosacea. N Engl J Med 2005;352(8):793–803.

45. Lee WJ, Jung JM, Won KH, et al. Clinical evaluation of 368 patients with nasal rosacea: subtype classification and grading of nasal rosacea. Dermatology 2015;230(2):177–83.

46. Sibenge S, Gawkrodger DJ. Rosacea: a study of clinical patterns, blood flow, and the role of Demodex folliculorum. J Am Acad Dermatol 1992;26(4):590–3.

47. Harvey DT, Fenske NA, Glass LF. Rosaceous lymphedema: a rare variant of a common disorder. Cutis 1998;61(6):321–4. Available at: http://www.ncbi.nlm.nih.gov/pubmed/9640553. Accessed January 15, 2017.

48. Knight AG, Vickers CF. A follow-up of tetracycline-treated rosacea. With special reference to rosacea keratitis. Br J Dermatol 1975;93(5):577–80. Available at: http://www.ncbi.nlm.nih.gov/pubmed/128376. Accessed January 18, 2017.

49. Dahl MV, Katz HI, Krueger GG, et al. Topical metronidazole maintains remissions of rosacea. Arch Dermatol 1998;134(6):679–83.

50. Wilkin JK. Use of topical products for maintaining remission in rosacea. Arch Dermatol 1999;135(1):79–80. Available at: http://www.ncbi.nlm.nih.gov/pubmed/9923787. Accessed January 18, 2017.

51. Olazagasti J, Lynch P, Fazel N. The great mimickers of rosacea. Cutis 2014;94(1):39–45. Available at: http://www.ncbi.nlm.nih.gov/pubmed/25101343. Accessed January 15, 2017.

52. Wilkin JK. Flushing reactions in the cancer chemotherapy patient. Arch Dermatol 1992;128(10):1387.

53. Greaves MW, Burova EP. Flushing: causes, investigation and clinical consequences. J Eur Acad Dermatol Venereol 1997;8(2):91–100.

54. Williams RE, Kalilani L, DiBenedetti DB, et al. Frequency and severity of vasomotor symptoms among peri- and postmenopausal women in the United States. Climacteric 2008;11(1):32–43.

55. Creamer JD, Whittaker SJ, Griffiths WA. Multiple endocrine neoplasia type 1 presenting as rosacea. Clin Exp Dermatol 1996;21(2):170–1. Available at: http://www.ncbi.nlm.nih.gov/pubmed/8759212. Accessed February 19, 2017.

56. Reichert S, Truchetet F, Cuny JF, et al. [Carcinoid tumor with revealed by skin manifestation]. Ann Dermatol Venereol 1994;121(6–7):485–8. Available at: http://www.ncbi.nlm.nih.gov/pubmed/7535513. Accessed February 19, 2017.

57. Findlay GH, Simson IW. Leonine hypertrophic rosacea associated with a benign bronchial carcinoid tumour. Clin Exp Dermatol 1977;2(2):175–6. Available at: http://www.ncbi.nlm.nih.gov/pubmed/195761. Accessed February 19, 2017.

58. Izikson L, English JC, Zirwas MJ. The flushing patient: differential diagnosis, workup, and treatment. J Am Acad Dermatol 2006;55(2):193–208.

59. Bell HK, Poston GJ, Vora J, et al. Cutaneous manifestations of the malignant carcinoid syndrome. Br J Dermatol 2005;152(1):71–5.

60. Wilkin JK. Erythematotelangiectatic rosacea and telangiectatic photoaging. JAMA Dermatol 2015; 151(8):821.

61. Helfrich YR, Maier LE, Cui Y, et al. Clinical, histologic, and molecular analysis of differences between erythematotelangiectatic rosacea and telangiectatic photoaging. JAMA Dermatol 2015;151(8):825.

62. Oldenburg M, Kuechmeister B, Ohnemus U, et al. Extrinsic skin ageing symptoms in seafarers subject to high work-related exposure to UV radiation. Eur J Dermatol 2013;23(5):663–70.

63. Berg M. Epidemiological studies of the influence of sunlight on the skin. Photodermatology 1989;6(2): 80–4. Available at: http://www.ncbi.nlm.nih.gov/pubmed/2748434. Accessed January 30, 2017.

64. Leyden JJ. Clinical features of ageing skin. Br J Dermatol 1990;122(Suppl 35):1–3. Available at: http://www.ncbi.nlm.nih.gov/pubmed/2186777. Accessed January 15, 2017.

65. Gilchrest BA. A review of skin ageing and its medical therapy. Br J Dermatol 1996;135(6):867–75.

66. Gilchrest BA. Skin aging and photoaging: an overview. J Am Acad Dermatol 1989;21(3 Pt 2):610–3.

67. Wilkin JK. Rosacea: pathophysiology and treatment. Arch Dermatol 1994;130(3):359–62.

68. Danby FW. Rosacea, acne rosacea, and actinic telangiectasia. J Am Acad Dermatol 2005;52(3): 539–40.

69. Stern RS. Treatment of photoaging. N Engl J Med 2004;350(15):1526–34.

70. Ramos-e-Silva M, Pirmez R. Red face revisited: disorders of hair growth and the pilosebaceous unit. Clin Dermatol 2014;32(6):784–99.

71. Rebora A. Periorbital lesions. Clin Dermatol 2011; 29(2):151–6.

72. Kazandjieva J, Tsankov N, Pramatarov K. The red face revisited: connective tissue disorders. Clin Dermatol 2014;32(1):153–8.

73. Okiyama N, Kohsaka H, Ueda N, et al. Seborrheic area erythema as a common skin manifestation in Japanese patients with dermatomyositis. Dermatology 2008;217(4):374–7.

74. Brown TT, Choi EY, Thomas DG, et al. Comparative analysis of rosacea and cutaneous lupus erythematosus: histopathologic features, T-cell subsets, and plasmacytoid dendritic cells. J Am Acad Dermatol 2014;71(1):1–8.

A Review of the Current Modalities for the Treatment of Papulopustular Rosacea

Sean P. McGregor, DO, PharmD[a], Hossein Alinia, MD[a],*,
Alyson Snyder, DO[a], Sara Moradi Tuchayi, MD, MPH[a],
Alan Fleischer Jr, MD[a], Steven R. Feldman, MD, PhD[a,b,c]

KEYWORDS

- Doxycycline • Metronidazole • Azelaic acid • Ivermectin • Topical • Management • Papulopustular
- Rosacea

KEY POINTS

- Rosacea is an inflammatory skin disorder that is characterized by a wide variety of clinical manifestations.
- Topical and oral antimicrobials are the mainstay of therapy for the treatment of papulopustular rosacea.
- This article highlights the current literature surrounding the treatment of papulopustular rosacea and aims to help clinicians in making treatment decisions in clinical practice.

INTRODUCTION

Rosacea is a common inflammatory skin disorder. It is classically seen in patients with lighter skin types, and the National Rosacea Society Expert Committee divides rosacea into 4 subtypes.[1,2] The papulopustular subtype of rosacea is characterized by the presence of persistent central facial erythema, in addition to inflammatory papules and pustules, which are transient in nature.[2] Phymatous changes and ocular manifestations may exist alone or in conjunction with papulopustular rosacea (PPR). In addition to these findings, patients often complain of dryness, burning, and stinging sensations in affected areas.[3,4] Topical and oral antimicrobials are the mainstay of therapy for the

Disclosure Statement: S.P. McGregor, H. Alinia, S.M. Tuchayi, and A. Snyder have nothing to disclose. S.R. Feldman is a speaker for Janssen and Taro. He is a consultant and speaker for Galderma, Stiefel/GlaxoSmithKline, Abbott Labs, and Leo Pharma. Inc. S.R. Feldman has received grants from Galderma, Janssen, Abbott Labs, Amgen, Stiefel, GlaxoSmithKline, Celgene, and Anacor. He is a consultant for Amgen, Baxter, Caremark, Gerson Lehrman Group, Guidepoint Global, Hanall Pharmaceutical Co Ltd, Kikaku, Lilly, Merck & Co Inc, Merz Pharmaceuticals, Mylan, Novartis Pharmaceuticals, Pfizer Inc, Qurient, Suncare Research, and Xenoport. He is on an advisory board for Pfizer Inc. S.R. Feldman is the founder of and holds stock in Causa Research, and holds stock and is majority owner in Medical Quality Enhancement Corporation. He receives Royalties from UpToDate and Xlibris. A. Fleischer Jr has received support for research, speaking, or consulting from Abbvie, Galderma, Regeneron, Eli Lilly, and Celgene and is employed by Merz Pharmaceuticals.
[a] Department of Dermatology, Center for Dermatology Research, Wake Forest School of Medicine, Medical Center Boulevard, Winston-Salem, NC 27157-1071, USA; [b] Department of Pathology, Wake Forest School of Medicine, Medical Center Boulevard, Winston-Salem, NC 27157-1071, USA; [c] Department of Public Health Sciences, Wake Forest School of Medicine, Medical Center Boulevard, Winston-Salem, NC 27157-1071, USA
* Corresponding author. Department of Dermatology, Wake Forest School of Medicine, Medical Center Boulevard, Winston-Salem, NC 27157-1071.
E-mail address: haliniamd@gmail.com

Dermatol Clin 36 (2018) 135–150
https://doi.org/10.1016/j.det.2017.11.009

treatment of PPR, and numerous clinical trials comparing efficacy, tolerability, and quality of life measures have been performed. The primary objective of this article is to review the current literature pertaining to the treatment of PPR and to provide evidence-based recommendations regarding the appropriate management of rosacea.

METHODS

A PubMed search of articles published from 1980 to 2015 was performed using the following MeSH terms: rosacea and clinical trial. EMBASE and the Cochrane (Central) databases were searched using the keywords, "rosacea" and "clinical trial." After the initial search was performed, additional searches were performed to include rosacea and each treatment modality used. The abstracts of each article were screened; studies on erythematotelangiectatic, phymatous, and ocular rosacea were excluded. Trials with fewer than 10 subjects, and those not in English were excluded. The remaining articles were reviewed for objective measures of efficacy. Articles that studied steroid rosacea or non–efficacy-related outcomes were excluded. Studies primarily assessing patient perspective quality of life and not objective measures of improvement were excluded. Articles with primary and secondary endpoints related to the Investigator's Global Assessment (IGA), Physician's Global Assessment, erythema severity, and inflammatory lesion count (ILC) were included in the review (**Fig. 1**). A table including trials meeting criteria was developed and scored based on the JADAD criteria.[5]

RESULTS

A total of 154 articles were identified after the initial search. A total of 52 articles were excluded owing to non-English language or subject matter. A total of 102 articles were reviewed in entirety, 66 articles that studied steroid rosacea, quality of life, non–efficacy-related outcomes, or had incomparable data were excluded (see **Fig. 1, Table 1**). A total of 36 articles were included in the final analysis. Owing to the lack of standardization among clinical trial results, we were unable to develop a true comparative statistical analysis. Variation with regard to ILC reduction and/or change in IGA was reported in some trials (see **Table 1**). Most trials either reported the percent reduction in ILC or the true reduction in ILC without a standard deviation or 95% confidence interval.

Doxycycline

Tetracycline antibiotics have been used for more than 60 years, and modified-release doxycycline

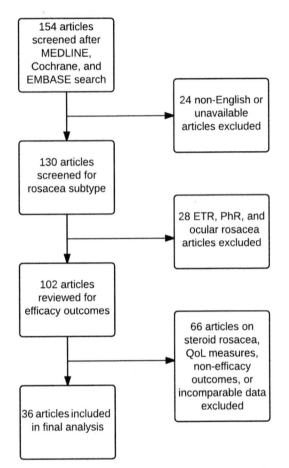

Fig. 1. Results of literature search regarding papulopustular rosacea. ETR, erythematotelangiectatic rosacea; PhR, phymatous rosacea; QoL, quality of life.

40 mg orally once daily is the only systemic agent approved by the US Food and Drug Administration for the treatment of PPR.[41,42] In PPR, the goal is to achieve subantimicrobial dosing and antiinflammatory effects that reduces the number of inflammatory lesions and limits adverse effects. Cost and individual patient pharmacokinetics may preclude the exclusive use of modified-release doxycycline. Doxycycline is the most well-studied tetracycline antibiotic for the treatment of PPR, and its efficacy is well-documented in clinical trials.[8–12,21] Doses of 40 to 200 mg daily are routinely used in clinical practice. Higher doses of doxycycline may be devoid of additional benefit and are accompanied by an increased risk of adverse effects.[10] A study that compared doxycycline 40 mg daily with 100 mg daily found no difference with regard to overall benefit, but an increased risk of nausea, vomiting, diarrhea, and abdominal pain associated with higher doses.[10] The risk of phototoxicity and pill esophagitis increase when using

Table 1
Comparison of studies in PPR

Authors	Patients (n)	Medication	Study Type	Duration	Results	JADAD Score
Stein Gold et al,[6] 2014 (2 studies)	Moderate-to-severe PPR (n = 683, 688) IGA score 3–4 ILC = 15–70	IVM 1% cream daily	R, DB, VC	12 wk	IGA score clear or almost clear = 38.4%, P<.05 Mean reduction in ILC = 76% IGA score clear or almost clear = 40.1%, P<.05 Mean reduction in ILC = −75%	5 5
Taieb et al,[7] 2015	Moderate-to-severe PPR (n = 926) IGA score 3–4 ILC = 15–70	IVM 1% cream daily vs MTZ 0.75% cream BID	R, SB, AC	16 wk	IGA score clear or almost clear = 84.9% vs 75.4%, P<.001 Mean reduction in ILC = −83% vs 73.7%, P<.001	4
Webster,[8] 2010	Mild-to-severe PPR (n = 1197) IGA score 2–4 CEA score 2–4	Doxycycline 40 mg PO daily	OL, O	12 wk	IGA score clear or almost clear = 74.6%, P<.0001 CEA score none (0) or mild (1) = 74.5%, P<.0001	1
Del Rosso,[9] 2010	Mild-to-severe PPR on topical MTZ, AzA, or SS (n = 224) IGA score 2–4 CEA score 2–4	Doxycycline 40 mg PO daily	OL, O	12 wk	IGA score clear or almost clear = 75.7%, P = .0012 CEA score mild (1) = 63.6%, P = .0407	1
Del Rosso et al,[10] 2008	Moderate-to-very severe PPR (n = 91) IGA score 2–5 Erythema score 5–20 with 1 area CEA ≥2 ILC = 8–40	Doxycycline 40 mg PO daily and MTZ 1% gel daily vs doxycycline 100 mg PO daily and MTZ 1% gel daily	R, DB, AC	16 wk	Mean change in IGA = −1.6 vs −1.6 (P = .86) Mean change in CEA score = −4.2 vs −4.0 (P = .5) Mean change in ILC = −12.5 vs −12.2 (P = .83)	4

(continued on next page)

Table 1
(continued)

Authors	Patients (n)	Medication	Study Type	Duration	Results	JADAD Score
Del Rosso et al,[11] 2007 (2 studies)	Moderate-to-severe PPR (n = 251, 286) IGA 3–4 CEA score 2–4 ILC = 10–40	Doxycycline 40 mg PO daily	R, DB, PC	16 wk	IGA clear or almost clear = 30.7% ($P<.001$) Mean change in CEA score = −2.7 ($P = .17$) Mean change in ILC = −11.8 ($P<.001$) IGA clear or almost clear = 14.8% ($P = .012$) No significant difference in CEA scores Mean change in ILC = −9.5 ($P<.001$)	5 5
Fowler,[12] 2007	Moderate-to-very severe PPR (n = 72) IGA score 2–5 Erythema score 5–20 ILC = 8–40	Doxycycline 40 mg PO daily + MTZ 1% gel daily vs MTZ 1% gel daily	R, DB, PC	12 wk (4-wk extension)	Mean % change in IGA = −66.4% vs −48.2% ($P = .008$) Mean change in erythema score = −1.3 vs −0.8 ($P = .01$) Mean change in ILC = −13.86 vs −9.69 ($P = .002$)	3
Thiboutot et al,[13] 2003 (2 trials)	Moderate PPR (n = 329, 335) ILC = 8–50	AzA 15% gel BID	R, DB, VC	12 wk	IGA clear, almost clear, or mild = 61%, $P<.0001$ Improvement in erythema score = 44%, $P = .0017$ Mean % change in ILC = −58%, $P = .0001$ IGA clear, almost clear, or mild = 62%, $P = .0127$ Improvement in erythema score = 46%, $P = .0005$ Mean % change in ILC = −51%, $P = .0208$	4 4

Draelos et al,[14] 2013	Moderate-to-severe PPR (n = 401) IGA 3–4 ILC = 12–50	AzA 15% foam BID	R, DB, VC	16 wk	IGA clear or almost clear = 43.4% (P = .017) No significant difference in erythema Mean (SD) change in ILC = −13.4 ± 10.4 (P<.001) Mean % change in ILC = −64.5% (P<.001)	5
Thiboutot et al,[15] 2009	Moderate-to-severe PPR (n = 172) IGA ≥4 ILC ≥10	AzA 15% gel BID and doxycycline 100 mg PO BID	OL, O	12 wk	IGA clear, minimal, or mild = 64% No or mild erythema = 56.4% Mean % change in ILC = −82%	1
	Moderate-to-severe PPR (n = 136) Extension for patients with ≥75% reduction in ILC	AzA 15% gel BID	R, DB, VC	24 wk (extension)	IGA clear, minimal, or mild = 58.2% Worsening erythema = 17.9% Relapse rate of ILC = 19.4% vs 29%	3
Thiboutot et al,[16] 2008	Mild-to-moderate PPR (n = 72) ILC = 10–50	AzA 15% gel daily vs AzA 15% gel BID	R, DB, VC	12 wk	IGA clear or minimal 37.5% vs 40.5% (P = .7887) Decrease in intensity of erythema with no significant difference between groups (P = .966) Mean % change in ILC = 63.3% vs 71.1% (P = .3028)	4

(continued on next page)

Table 1
(continued)

Authors	Patients (n)	Medication	Study Type	Duration	Results	JADAD Score
Jackson et al,[17] 2014	Mild-to-severe PPR (n = 60) IGA 2–4 CEA ≥2 ILC = 10–40	Minocycline 40 mg ER PO daily vs AzA 15% daily and minocycline 40 mg ER PO daily	R, DB	12 wk (4 wk follow-up)	IGA clear or almost clear = 57% vs 60% (P = .5) Median (min, max) change in CEA score = −3 [−9, 6] vs −4 [−9, 3] (P = .49) Mean (SD) change in ILC = −11 ± 5 vs −12 ± 7 (P = .6)	4
Elewski et al,[18] 2003	Moderate PPR (n = 251) ILC = 10–50	AzA 15% gel BID vs MTZ 0.75% gel BID	R, DB, AC	15 wk	IGA clear, minimal, or mild 69% vs 55% (P = .02) Improvement in erythema severity = 56% vs 42% (P = .02) Mean change in ILC = −12.9 vs −10.7 (P = .003) Mean % change in ILC = 72.7% vs 55.8% (P<.001)	5
Maddin et al,[19] 1999	Mild-to-severe PPR (n = 40) ILC ≥10	AzA 20% cream BID vs MTZ 1% cream BID	R, DB, SF	15 wk	Approximately 50%–75% physician rating global improvement with no significant difference between groups Reduction in erythema = 39.5% vs 27% (P = .05) Mean % change in ILC = −78.5% vs 69.4% (P = .43)	3

Study	Population	Treatment	Design	Duration	Results	Quality
Del Rosso et al,[20] 2010	Mild-to-moderate PPR (n = 207) IGA ≥4 Persistent Erythema ILC = 10–50	AzA 15% gel BID and doxycycline 40 mg PO daily vs MTZ 1% gel daily and doxycycline 40 mg PO daily	R, SB, AC	2 wk (12 wk)	IGA clear, minimal, or mild = 78.3% vs 72.3% Mean change in ILC after 2 wk = −10.5 vs −9.4 ($P = .38$)	3
Sanchez et al,[21] 2005	Moderate-to-very severe PPR (n = 40) CGSS 2–4 Erythema score 2–4 CGEA 5–20 ILC = 8–30	Doxycycline 20 mg PO BID and MTZ 0.75% lotion BID vs Placebo and MTZ 0.75% lotion BID	R, DB, PC	12 wk (4 wk monotherapy with doxycycline)	Mean change in CGSS at 12 wk ≈ −1.0 vs −0.4 ($P = .046$) Mean change in CGSS at 16 wk ≈ −0.9 vs −0.4 No significant change in CGEA Mean change in ILC at 12 wk ≈ −16 vs −7 ($P<.01$) Mean change in ILC at 16 wk ≈ −15 vs −5 ($P<.01$)	5
Dahl et al,[22] 1998	Moderate-to-severe PPR (n = 113) Erythema score ≥2 ILC ≥6 Patients with >70% decrease in ILC (n = 88)	TCN 250 mg PO QID (tapered BID, QD, then off over 4 wk) and MTZ 0.75% gel BID	OL, O	16 wk	Reduction in erythema from moderate to mild Mean (SD) change in ILC = −13.6 ± 3.1	1
		MTZ 0.75% gel BID	DB, VC	24 wk (extension)	6-mo relapse-free interval = 77% ($P<.05$) Mild or no erythema = 74% Mean ILC = 3.3 vs 5.8 ($P<.01$)	3
Wolf & Del Rosso,[23] 2007	Mild-to-moderately severe PPR (n = 582) Mild-to-moderate erythema ≥ 1 mo ILC = 8–30	MTZ 0.75% gel BID	OL, O	12 wk	IGA clear or almost clear = 42% ($P<.0001$) Reduction in erythema = 45% ($P<.0001$) Mean % change in ILC = −71% ($P<.0001$)	1

(continued on next page)

Table 1
(continued)

Authors	Patients (n)	Medication	Study Type	Duration	Results	JADAD Score
Bleicher et al,[24] 1987	Moderate-to-severe PPR (n = 40) Moderate erythema ILC ≥3 on each side of face	MTZ 0.75% gel BID	R, DB, VC, SF	9 wk (12 wk)	Mean reduction in erythema score = 0.8, 0.6 (P = .0006, .0086) Mean % change in ILC = −65.1%(−48.1%)	4
Jorizzo et al,[25] 1998	Moderate-to-severe PPR (n = 227) Rosacea score ≥2	MTZ 1% cream daily vs MTZ 1% cream BID	R, DB, AC, VC	10 wk	PGA fair or better improvement = 79% vs 72% Reduction in erythema = −41% vs −36% Mean % change in ILC = −58% vs −58%	3
Dahl et al,[26] 2001	Moderate-to-severe PPR (n = 72) Total erythema score ≥7 or ≥2 from 2/5 regions ILC = 8–50	MTZ 0.75% cream daily vs MTZ 1% cream daily	R, SB, AC	12 wk	IGA clear or mild = 63% vs 45% (P≥.45) Reduction in erythema = 26% vs 30% (P≥.38) Mean % reduction in ILC = 62% vs 60% (P≥.29)	3
Torok et al,[27] 2005	Moderate-to-severe PPR (n = 152) IGS ≥ moderate Erythema ≥ moderate ILC = 10–39	Sodium sulfacetamide/sulfur 10/5% cream + sunscreen BID vs MTZ 0.75% cream BID	R, SB	12 wk	IGA of clear, excellent, or good = 79% vs 59% (P = .01) Improvement in erythema = 69% vs 45% (P = .0007) Mean % change in ILC = −80% vs −72% (P = .04)	3

Study	Population	Intervention	Design	Duration	Results	
Altinyazar et al,[28] 2013	PPR (n = 55) ILC ≥10	Adapalene 0.10% gel QHS vs MTZ 0.75% gel BID	R, SB, AC	12 wk	No significant change in erythema with adapalene; Mean change in erythema grade with MTZ ≈ −1.5 ($P<.05$); Mean change in ILC = −10.11 vs −9.32	3
Koca et al,[29] 2010	PPR (n = 49) ILC ≥10	MTZ 1% cream BID vs pimecrolimus 1% cream BID	R, OL, AC	12 wk	PGA complete clearance = 83.3% vs 48% ($P>.05$); Reduction in erythema = −45.8% vs −44.7% ($P = .23$); Mean % change in ILC = −97.3% vs −88.9% ($P = .55$)	3
Freeman et al,[30] 2012	Rosacea (n = 20) FST I-III Persistent central facial redness	Clindamycin 1.2% and Tretinoin 0.025% gel daily	R, DB, VC	12 wk	No significant difference in colorimetry measurements; Mean % change in ILC = −46%	3
Chang et al,[31] 2012	PPR (n = 83) ILC = 4–50	Clindamycin 1.2% and tretinoin 0.025% gel daily	R, DB, VC	12 wk	PGA improvement = 25% ($P = .58$); Erythema improvement = 28% ($P = .27$); Mean difference in ILC = 0.83 ± 10.84 ($P = .63$)	5
Breneman et al,[32] 2004	PPR (n =) ORSA ≥2.5 ILC = 8–50	Clindamycin 1%/BPO 5% gel daily	R, DB, VC	12 wk	PGA clear or marked improvement = 42.3% ($P = .0378$); Mean % ORSA improvement = 29.3% ($P = .01$); Mean % change in ILC = 71.3 ± 25.3% ($P<.0001$)	5

(continued on next page)

Table 1
(continued)

Authors	Patients (n)	Medication	Study Type	Duration	Results	JADAD Score
Ertl et al,[33] 1994	Severe, recalcitrant PPR	Tretinoin 0.025% cream daily vs isotretinoin 10 mg PO daily vs tretinoin 0.025% cream daily and isotretinoin 10 mg PO daily	R, DB, AC, PC, VC, CO	32 wk	Mean erythema score change = −27%, −40%, −41% Mean change in ILC = −5.6, −9.1, −11.9	4
Bamford et al,[34] 2004	ETR or PPR (n = 24)	Tacrolimus 0.1% ointment BID	OL, O	12 wk	No significant change in ILC	1
Kim et al,[35] 2011	Mild-to-moderate ETR or PPR (n = 30)	Pimecrolimus 1% cream BID	OL, O	4 wk	Mean change in RCS = −2.38 (P<.05) Mean change in IGA = 0.97 Significant reduction in IGA seen after 2 wk, no change at 4 wk	1
Karabulut et al,[36] 2008	PPR (n = 25)	Pimecrolimus 1% cream BID	R, SB, VC, SF	4 wk (2 wk)	Mean % reduction in RSS 95.83% vs 91.67% (P = .06)	3
Weissenbacher et al,[37] 2007	PPR (n = 40)	Pimecrolimus 1% cream BID	R, DB, VC	4-8 wk	Mean % improvement in RSS = 32% vs 37% (P = .39)	3
Schlesinger & Powell,[38] 2007	Mild-to-moderate rosacea (n = 14) FST I-IV	Hyaluronic acid 0.2% cream BID	OL, O	8 wk	Mean % improvement in PGA = 47.5% Mean % reduction in ILC = −47%	1

Study	Population	Treatment	Design	Duration	Outcome	Quality
Ortiz et al,[39] 2009	Mild-to-moderate ETR or PPR	PRK124 0.125% lotion BID	OL, O	12 wk	Mean % improvement in ILC ≈ 40%	1
Bamford et al,[40] 2012	Moderate-to-severe PPR (n = 53)	Zinc sulfate 220 mg BID	R, DB, PC	12 wk	Mean difference in RSS = 0.57 ($P = .284$) Stopper early owing to lack of benefit	4
Akhyani et al,[53] 2008	PPR (n = 67)	Azithromycin 500 mg PO Monday, Wednesday, Friday for 1 mo, 250 mg PO Monday, Wednesday, Friday for 1 mo, then 250 mg PO Tuesday and Saturday for 1 mo vs doxycycline 100 mg PO daily	R, OL	20 wk	Mean change in ILC = − 17.6 vs − 16.9 Mean % change in ILC = 91% vs 89%	3

Abbreviations: AC, active comparator; AzA, azelaic acid; BID, twice a day; BPO, benzoyl peroxide; CEA, Clinician's Erythema Assessment; CGEA, Clinician's Global Erythema Assessment; CGSS, Clinician's Global Severity Score; CO, crossover; DB, double blind; ER, extended release; ETR, erythematotelangiectatic rosacea; FST, Fitzpatrick skin type; IGA, Investigator's Global Assessment; ILC, inflammatory lesion count; IVM, ivermectin; IGS, Investigator's Global Severity; MTZ, metronidazole; O, observational; OL, open label; ORSA, Overall Rosacea Severity Assessment; PC, placebo-controlled; PGA, Physician's Global Assessment; PO, by mouth; PPR, papulopustular rosacea; QD, daily; QID, 4 times per day; R, randomized; RCS, rosacea clinical score (IGA scores vary from 0–4 to 0–7 depending on study); RSS, Rosacea Severity Score; SB, single blind; SD, standard deviation; SF, split face; SS, sodium sulfacetamide/sulfur; TCN, tetracycline; VC, vehicle-controlled.

higher doses and immediate release formulations, respectively. Doxycycline is generally safe and effective in the treatment of PPR.[10] Although doxycycline remains the tetracycline of choice in the treatment of PPR, extended-release minocycline provides similar reductions in ILC.[17] Minocycline may be a potential alternative for patients unresponsive to or intolerant of doxycycline (**Fig. 2**).

Topical Metronidazole

Topical metronidazole has been used successfully in the treatment of PPR for many years. Although its mechanism of action is yet to be fully elucidated, modulation of neutrophilic activity via reductions in reactive oxygen species is a common theory.[43] Metronidazole is available in concentrations of 1% and 0.75% for once or twice-daily application, respectively.[44] In clinical trials, topical metronidazole consistently reduced ILC and erythema, resulting in significantly improved investigator assessments.[23–26] Topical metronidazole is at least as effective as doxycycline for the treatment of PPR. Patient preference regarding topical versus oral treatment should be considered.[45] In patients with more severe disease, combination therapy with doxycycline and metronidazole provides added benefit, and continued topical application of metronidazole after discontinuation of doxycycline may maintain remission in approximately 80% of patients.[12,22] There is no difference in efficacy between once-daily or twice-daily application of the 1% formulation.[25] Although the 0.75% formulation is only approved for twice-daily application, it provides just as much clinical benefit when used daily in comparison with the 1% formulation.[26] Once-daily application of metronidazole may provide just as much clinical benefit as twice-daily application, with improved tolerability and adherence. Topical application of metronidazole is safe and well-tolerated. The most frequently observed adverse reactions include irritation and dermatitis.

Topical Azelaic Acid

Azelaic acid is available in two formulations, a 20% cream and a 15% gel. Only azelaic acid 15% gel is approved for the treatment of rosacea, but the 20% cream has been used successfully.[19] Azelaic acid is a dicarboxylic acid and its mechanism of action in rosacea is not fully understood. It is thought to reduce both kallikrein 5 expression and serine protease activity, two important components of the inflammatory cascade in rosacea.[44,46] Like topical metronidazole, azelaic acid produces significant reductions in ILC and comparable reductions in erythema.[13–16] In one study,

azelaic acid 15% gel produced significantly greater reductions in ILC and improvements in both erythema and IGA scores compared to metronidazole 0.75% gel.[18] However, a study that compared metronidazole 1% cream with azelaic acid 20% cream found no differences between major endpoints.[19] This discrepancy may be related to better solubility and penetration of the gel formulation compared to the cream.[47] With regard to tolerability, azelaic acid use is associated with facial irritation, dryness, and transient neurosensory sensations of stinging and burning.[48] Azelaic acid 15% gel is more efficacious than metronidazole 0.75%, but at the expense of greater toxicity.[49] However, there are no significant differences between azelaic acid 15% gel and metronidazole 1% with regard to efficacy and tolerability. Once-daily application of azelaic acid is as effective as twice-daily application and may be a suitable means to improve tolerability and adherence.[16]

Topical Ivermectin

Ivermectin is an antiparasitic agent that has been used orally for many years. Its mechanism of action in rosacea is unknown, but may be related to reductions in tumor necrosis factor-alpha and interleukin-1b.[50] Ivermectin is an effective agent against *Demodex* mites, which may be implicated in the underlying pathophysiology of rosacea.[51] In two clinical trials, treatment with ivermectin 1% cream revealed significant reductions in ILC and improvements in IGA scores compared to vehicle.[6] One study that compared once-daily application of ivermectin 1% cream with twice-daily application of metronidazole 0.75% cream noted greater reductions in ILC and improvement in IGA scores with ivermectin.[7] Patient-reported outcomes and quality of life measures were better with ivermectin in comparison with metronidazole.[7] The most commonly reported adverse effects with ivermectin use are similar to metronidazole and azelaic acid and include irritation, xerosis, burning, and pruritus. In a 40-week trial comparing the tolerability of ivermectin with that of azelaic acid, approximately 2% of patients in the ivermectin group and 6% of patients in the azelaic acid group experienced drug-related adverse effects.[6] Topical ivermectin is safe, and more efficacious than topical metronidazole, in moderate-to-severe disease. Once-daily application may improve adherence in comparison with twice-daily regimens.

Other Agents

A number of other agents have been studied in patients with PPR, all of which have relatively mixed

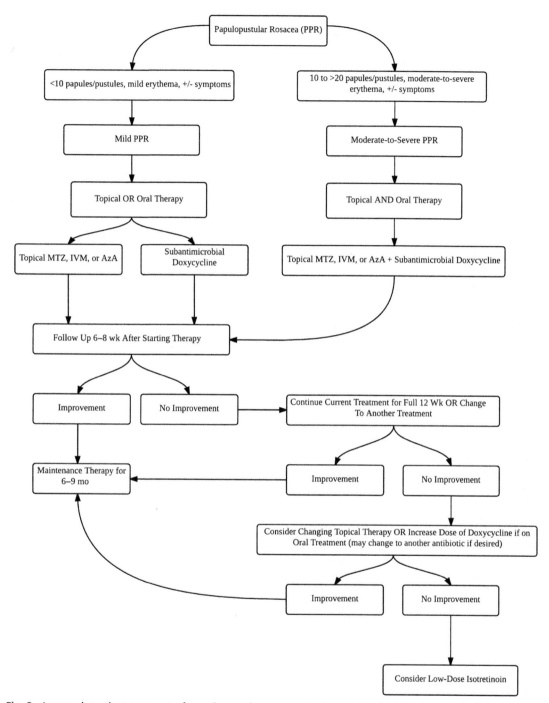

Fig. 2. Approach to the treatment of papulopustular rosacea. AzA, azelaic acid; IVM, ivermectin; MTZ, metronidazole; PPR, papulopustular rosacea. *Data from* Two AM, Wu W, Gallo RL, et al. Rosacea: Part II. Topical and
systemic therapies in the treatment of rosacea. J Am Acad Dermatol 2015;72(5):761–70; and Del Rosso JQ,
Thiboutot D, Gallo R, et al. American Acne & Rosacea Society. Consensus recommendations from the American
Acne & Rosacea Society on the management of rosacea, part 5: a guide on the management of rosacea Cutis
2014;93(3):134–8.

results. Sodium sulfacetamide/sulfur 10/5% cream with sunscreen reduced ILC and improved erythema and rosacea severity in comparison with topical metronidazole.[27] Adverse effects, such as burning, irritation, and a foul smell are substantial drawbacks to its use. Because sun exposure may exacerbate rosacea, the addition of sunscreen to sodium sulfacetamide/sulfur in this regimen may have confounded the results.

Topical clindamycin, tretinoin, and calcineurin inhibitors, such as tacrolimus and pimecrolimus, have been studied in PPR. However, none of these modalities provided any substantial benefit over placebo.[30–37] Oral isotretinoin at 10 mg daily was effective in reducing ILC and erythema in patients with severe, recalcitrant rosacea.[33] Oral macrolide antibiotics, such as azithromycin, in various doses have been studied in PPR, but inconsistent results, gastrointestinal adverse effects, and the potential for macrolide resistance are limitations to their use.[52–54] However, azithromycin may be a suitable option for patients who are unable to take doxycycline, such as pregnant women (see **Table 1**, see **Fig. 2**).

DISCUSSION

Rosacea is a chronic disorder with tremendous psychosocial impact. Embarrassment, reduced self-esteem, and decreased quality of life are all factors that should be considered when treating patients with rosacea. Statistically and clinically significant improvements in IGA scores correlate to improvements in quality of life.[55]

Topical metronidazole, azelaic acid, ivermectin, and oral doxycycline have the most robust data to support their use. Variation in assessment tools and a lack of standardization among clinical trials makes comparison of therapeutic options difficult. The lack of a comparative statistical analysis between each treatment is a significant limitation of this study.[56] A Cochrane review of interventions for rosacea revealed that topical azelaic acid, topical ivermectin, doxycycline, and isotretinoin have the highest quality of evidence in support of efficacy.[57] The results of this review are consistent with those findings.

SUMMARY

The management of rosacea is complex and multifactorial, requiring an individualized approach. Patients with primarily centrofacial erythema and papulopustular lesions are often treated with topical therapy alone or a combination of oral and topical therapy based on the severity[45] (see **Fig. 2**). In this review, we provide clinicians with an evidence-based approach to the management of rosacea. There may be overlap between each subtype of rosacea, and patients often present with a multitude of findings not strictly limited to PPR. This factor is problematic because reductions in ILC provide us with only one objective measure of efficacy and do not take into account reductions in erythema or other rosacea symptomatology. Likewise, individual patient characteristics should always be taken into consideration when managing rosacea, and other therapeutic modalities may need to be used if significant erythema, telangiectasias, and phymatous changes are of concern. The results of this study do not address these concerns. This issue is important, because quality randomized controlled trials in rosacea are lacking and clinicians may need to use various modalities to achieve success. Overall, the results of this review are consistent with the current American Acne and Rosacea Society guidelines. Inclusion of data on topical ivermectin provides dermatologists with the most up-to-date, evidence-based approach to the management of PPR[45] (see **Fig. 2**).

REFERENCES

1. Spoendlin J, Voegel JJ, Jick SS, et al. A study on the epidemiology of rosacea in the U.K. Br J Dermatol 2012;167(3):598–605.
2. Wilkin J, Dahl M, Detmar M, et al. Standard classification of rosacea: report of the national rosacea society expert committee on the classification and staging of rosacea. J Am Acad Dermatol 2002; 46(4):584–7.
3. Tan J, Berg M. Rosacea: current state of epidemiology. J Am Acad Dermatol 2013;69(6 Suppl 1): S27–35.
4. Del Rosso JQ. Management of cutaneous rosacea: emphasis on new medical therapies. Expert Opin Pharmacother 2014;15(14):2029–38.
5. Jadad AR, Moore RA, Carroll D, et al. Assessing the quality of reports of randomized clinical trials: is blinding necessary? Control Clin Trials 1996;17(1): 1–12.
6. Stein L, Kircik L, Fowler J, et al. Efficacy and safety of ivermectin 1% cream in treatment of papulopustular rosacea: results of two randomized, double-blind, vehicle-controlled pivotal studies. J Drugs Dermatol 2014;13(3):316–23.
7. Taieb A, Ortonne JP, Ruzicka T, et al. Ivermectin phase III study group. Superiority of ivermectin 1% cream over metronidazole 0·75% cream in treating inflammatory lesions of rosacea: a randomized, investigator-blinded trial. Br J Dermatol 2015; 172(4):1103–10.

8. Webster GF. An open-label, community-based, 12-week assessment of the effectiveness and safety of monotherapy with doxycycline 40 mg (30-mg immediate-release and 10-mg delayed-release beads). Cutis 2010;86(5 Suppl):7–15.

9. Del Rosso JQ. Effectiveness and safety of doxycycline 40 mg (30-mg immediate-release and 10-mg delayed-release beads) once daily as add-on therapy to existing topical regimens for the treatment of papulopustular rosacea: results from a community-based trial. Cutis 2010;86(5 Suppl):16–25.

10. Del Rosso JQ, Schlessinger J, Werschler P. Comparison of anti-inflammatory dose: doxycycline versus doxycycline 100 mg in the treatment of rosacea. J Drugs Dermatol 2008;7(6):573–6.

11. Del Rosso JQ, Webster GF, Jackson M, et al. Two randomized phase III clinical trials evaluating anti-inflammatory dose doxycycline (40-mg doxycycline, USP capsules) administered once daily for treatment of rosacea. J Am Acad Dermatol 2007;56(5):791–802.

12. Fowler JF Jr. Combined effect of anti-inflammatory dose doxycycline (40-mg doxycycline, USP monohydrate controlled-release capsules) and metronidazole topical gel 1% in the treatment of rosacea. J Drugs Dermatol 2007;6(6):641–5.

13. Thiboutot D, Thieroff-Ekerdt R, Graupe K. Efficacy and safety of azelaic acid (15%) gel as a new treatment for papulopustular rosacea: results from two vehicle-controlled, randomized phase III studies. J Am Acad Dermatol 2003;48(6):836–45.

14. Draelos ZD, Elewski B, Staedtler G, et al. Azelaic acid foam 15% in the treatment of papulopustular rosacea: a randomized, double-blind, vehicle-controlled study. Cutis 2013;92(6):306–17.

15. Thiboutot DM, Fleischer AB, Del Rosso JQ, et al. A multicenter study of topical azelaic acid 15% gel in combination with oral doxycycline as initial therapy and azelaic acid 15% gel as maintenance monotherapy. J Drugs Dermatol 2009;8(7):639–48.

16. Thiboutot DM, Fleischer AB Jr, Del Rosso JQ, et al. Azelaic acid 15% gel once daily versus twice daily in papulopustular rosacea. J Drugs Dermatol 2008;7(6):541–6.

17. Jackson JM, Kircik LH, Lorenz DJ. Efficacy of extended-release 45 mg oral minocycline and extended-release 45 mg oral minocycline plus 15% azelaic acid in the treatment of acne rosacea. J Drugs Dermatol 2013;12(3):292–8.

18. Elewski BE, Fleischer AB Jr, Pariser DM. A comparison of 15% azelaic acid gel and 0.75% metronidazole gel in the topical treatment of papulopustular rosacea: results of a randomized trial. Arch Dermatol 2003;139(11):1444–50.

19. Maddin S. A comparison of topical azelaic acid 20% cream and topical metronidazole 0.75% cream in the treatment of patients with papulopustular rosacea. J Am Acad Dermatol 1999;40(6 Pt 1):961–5.

20. Del Rosso JQ, Bruce S, Jarratt M, et al. Efficacy of topical azelaic acid (AzA) gel 15% plus oral doxycycline 40 mg versus metronidazole gel 1% plus oral doxycycline 40 mg in mild-to-moderate papulopustular rosacea. J Drugs Dermatol 2010;9(6):607–13.

21. Sanchez J, Somolinos AL, Almodóvar PI, et al. A randomized, double-blind, placebo-controlled trial of the combined effect of doxycycline hyclate 20-mg tablets and metronidazole 0.75% topical lotion in the treatment of rosacea. J Am Acad Dermatol 2005;53(5):791–7.

22. Dahl MV, Katz HI, Krueger GG, et al. Topical metronidazole maintains remissions of rosacea. Arch Dermatol 1998;134(6):679–83.

23. Wolf JE Jr, Del Rosso JQ. The CLEAR trial: results of a large community-based study of metronidazole gel in rosacea. Cutis 2007;79(1):73–80.

24. Bleicher PA, Charles JH, Sober AJ. Topical metronidazole therapy for rosacea. Arch Dermatol 1987;123(5):609–14.

25. Jorizzo JL, Lebwohl M, Tobey RE. The efficacy of metronidazole 1% cream once daily compared with metronidazole 1% cream twice daily and their vehicles in rosacea: a double-blind clinical trial. J Am Acad Dermatol 1998;39(3):502–4.

26. Dahl MV, Jarratt M, Kaplan D, et al. Once-daily topical metronidazole cream formulations in the treatment of the papules and pustules of rosacea. J Am Acad Dermatol 2001;45(5):723–30.

27. Torok HM, Webster G, Dunlap FE, et al. Combination sodium sulfacetamide 10% and sulfur 5% cream with sunscreens versus metronidazole 0.75% cream for rosacea. Cutis 2005;75(6):357–63.

28. Altinyazar HC, Koca R, Tekin NS, et al. Adapalene vs. metronidazole gel for the treatment of rosacea. Int J Dermatol 2005;44(3):252–5.

29. Koca R, Altinyazar HC, Ankarali H, et al. A comparison of metronidazole 1% cream and pimecrolimus 1% cream in the treatment of patients with papulopustular rosacea: a randomized open-label clinical trial. Clin Exp Dermatol 2010;35(3):251–6.

30. Freeman SA, Moon SD, Spencer JM. Clindamycin phosphate 1.2% and tretinoin 0.025% gel for rosacea: summary of a placebo-controlled, double-blind trial. J Drugs Dermatol 2012;11(12):1410–4.

31. Chang AL, Alora-Palli M, Lima XT, et al. A randomized, double-blind, placebo-controlled, pilot study to assess the efficacy and safety of clindamycin 1.2% and tretinoin 0.025% combination gel for the treatment of acne rosacea over 12 weeks. J Drugs Dermatol 2012;11(3):333–9.

32. Breneman D, Savin R, VandePol C, et al. Double-blind, randomized, vehicle-controlled clinical trial of once-daily benzoyl peroxide/clindamycin topical gel in the treatment of patients with moderate to severe rosacea. Int J Dermatol 2004;43(5):381–7.

33. Ertl GA, Levine N, Kligman AM. A comparison of the efficacy of topical tretinoin and low-dose oral isotretinoin in rosacea. Arch Dermatol 1994;130(3):319–24.

34. Bamford JT, Elliott BA, Haller IV. Tacrolimus effect on rosacea. J Am Acad Dermatol 2004;50(1):107–8.

35. Kim MB, Kim GW, Park HJ, et al. Pimecrolimus 1% cream for the treatment of rosacea. J Dermatol 2011;38(12):1135–9.

36. Karabulut AA, Izol Serel B, Eksioglu HM. A randomized, single-blind, placebo-controlled, split-face study with pimecrolimus cream 1% for papulopustular rosacea. J Eur Acad Dermatol Venereol 2008;22(6):729–34.

37. Weissenbacher S, Merkl J, Hildebrandt B, et al. Pimecrolimus cream 1% for papulopustular rosacea: a randomized vehicle-controlled double-blind trial. Br J Dermatol 2007;156(4):728–32.

38. Schlesinger TE, Powell CR. Efficacy and tolerability of low molecular weight hyaluronic acid sodium salt 0.2% cream in rosacea. J Drugs Dermatol 2013;12(6):664–7.

39. Ortiz A, Elkeeb L, Truitt A, et al. 124 (0.125%) lotion for improving the signs and symptoms of rosacea. J Drugs Dermatol 2009;8(5):459–62.

40. Bamford JT, Gessert CE, Haller IV, et al. Randomized, double-blind trial of 220 mg zinc sulfate twice daily in the treatment of rosacea. Int J Dermatol 2012;51(4):459–62.

41. Del Rosso JQ, Thiboutot D, Gallo R, et al. Consensus recommendations from the American Acne & Rosacea Society on the management of rosacea, part 3: a status report on systemic therapies. Cutis 2014;93(1):18–28.

42. Two AM, Wu W, Gallo RL, et al. Rosacea: part II. Topical and systemic therapies in the treatment of rosacea. J Am Acad Dermatol 2015;72(5):761–70.

43. Narayanan S, Hünerbein A, Getie M, et al. Scavenging properties of metronidazole on free oxygen radicals in a skin lipid model system. J Pharm Pharmacol 2007;59(8):1125–30.

44. Del Rosso JQ, Thiboutot D, Gallo R, et al. Consensus recommendations from the American Acne & Rosacea Society on the management of rosacea, part 2: a status report on topical agents. Cutis 2013;92(6):277–84.

45. Del Rosso JQ, Thiboutot D, Gallo R, et al, American Acne & Rosacea Society. Consensus recommendations from the American Acne & Rosacea Society on

the management of rosacea, part 5: a guide on the management of rosacea. Cutis 2014;93(3):134–8.

46. Coda AB, Hata T, Miller J, et al. Cathelicidin, kallikrein 5, and serine protease activity is inhibited during treatment of rosacea with azelaic acid 15% gel. J Am Acad Dermatol 2013;69(4):570–7.

47. Draelos ZD. The rationale for advancing the formulation of azelaic acid vehicles. Cutis 2006;77(2 Suppl):7–11 [Review].

48. Draelos ZD. Noxious sensory perceptions in patients with mild to moderate rosacea treated with azelaic acid 15% gel. Cutis 2004;74(4):257–60.

49. Colón LE, Johnson LA, Gottschalk RW. Cumulative irritation potential among metronidazole gel 1%, metronidazole gel 0.75%, and azelaic acid gel 15%. Cutis 2007;79(4):317–21.

50. Ci X, Li H, Yu Q, et al. Avermectin exerts anti-inflammatory effect by downregulating the nuclear transcription factor kappa-B and mitogen-activated protein kinase activation pathway. Fundam Clin Pharmacol 2009;23(4):449–55.

51. O'Reilly N, Menezes N, Kavanagh K. Positive correlation between serum immunoreactivity to Demodex-associated Bacillus proteins and erythematotelangiectatic rosacea. Br J Dermatol 2012;167(5):1032–6.

52. Bakar O, Demirçay Z, Gürbüz O. Therapeutic potential of azithromycin in rosacea. Int J Dermatol 2004;43(2):151–4.

53. Akhyani M, Ehsani AH, Ghiasi M, et al. Comparison of efficacy azithromycin vs. doxycycline in the treatment of rosacea: a randomized open clinical trial. Int J Dermatol 2008;47(3):284–8.

54. Elewski BE. A novel treatment for acne vulgaris and rosacea. J Eur Acad Dermatol Venereol 2000;14(5):423–4.

55. Fleischer A, Suephy C. The face and mind evaluation study: an examination of the efficacy of rosacea treatment using physician ratings and patients' self-reported quality of life. J Drugs Dermatol 2005;4(5):585–90.

56. Hopkinson D, Moradi Tuchayi S, Alinia H, et al. Assessment of rosacea severity: a review of evaluation methods used in clinical trials. J Am Acad Dermatol 2015;73(1):138–43.e4.

57. van Zuuren EJ, Fedorowicz Z, Carter B, et al. Interventions for rosacea. Cochrane Database Syst Rev 2015;4:CD003262.

Medical Management of Facial Redness in Rosacea

Abigail Cline, MD, PhD[a], Sean P. McGregor, DO, PharmD[b],*, Steven R. Feldman, MD, PhD[b,c,d]

KEYWORDS

• Erythema • Topical • Management • Erythematotelangiectatic • Papulopustular • Rosacea

KEY POINTS

• Rosacea is a chronic skin condition characterized by central facial erythema and flushing.
• Options for the medical management of facial erythema, telangiectasias, and flushing are limited.
• Medications to reduce erythema and flushing may provide temporary relief but do not alter the chronic nature of the disease.
• The goal of this article is to review the topical and systemic treatments for rosacea-related erythema and flushing to help facilitate decision making in clinical practice.

INTRODUCTION

Rosacea is a chronic skin condition that presents with a broad diversity of cutaneous manifestations. Facial erythema, the most common primary characteristic of all subtypes of rosacea, is a mandatory diagnostic feature.[1,2] Persistent centrofacial erythema is the predominant hallmark of patients with rosacea, especially in the erythematotelangiectatic rosacea (ETR) and the papulopustular rosacea (PPR) subtypes.[3] Treatment has been difficult because, until recently, there were no effective medications for the erythema and flushing associated with rosacea.[4,5]

As with most chronic skin diseases, rosacea management requires long-term treatment with multiple modalities. Management strategies for people with rosacea should be tailored to the specific subtype of rosacea. For patients with mild symptoms, nonpharmacologic measures may be sufficient for reducing facial redness, flushing, skin sensitivity, and skin dryness. Successful rosacea management may be possible through avoidance of triggers that cause flushing, such as spicy foods, alcohol, exercise, sunlight, and some types of cosmetics.[6] When satisfactory improvement is not achieved through these lifestyle modifications, treatment with topical and systemic medications is an option.

New insights into the pathophysiology have led to advances in the management of rosacea. A deeper understanding of rosacea means more opportunities to target specific pathogenic factors and clinical manifestations with novel agents. Although topical metronidazole and azelaic acid and systemic tetracyclines are efficacious for PPR, there are few treatment options for persistent facial erythema.[7]

Novel treatments are on the horizon for the management of facial erythema of rosacea. Although it is unlikely that a single modality will result in complete and permanent resolution, treatment options are available that yield good results when tailored to the right clinical scenario. Topical medications, either as monotherapy or as part of a combination regimen, are the first-line choice and often sufficient for patients with mild to moderate ETR or

Disclosure: See last page of article.
[a] Augusta University Medical Center, Augusta, GA 30912, USA; [b] Center for Dermatology Research, Department of Dermatology, Wake Forest School of Medicine, Medical Center Boulevard, Winston-Salem, NC 27157-1071, USA; [c] Department of Pathology, Wake Forest School of Medicine, Winston-Salem, NC, USA; [d] Department of Public Health Sciences, Wake Forest School of Medicine, Winston-Salem, NC, USA
* Corresponding author.
E-mail address: smcgrego@wakehealth.edu

Dermatol Clin 36 (2018) 151–159
https://doi.org/10.1016/j.det.2017.11.010

PPR. Topical medications primarily used for PPR (eg, topical antimicrobials and azelaic acid) may also reduce rosacea-associated facial erythema.[8–10] However, telangiectasias are unlikely to improve with topicals and are best managed with light-based treatments. The authors discuss topical and systemic treatments for rosacea-related erythema and aim to facilitate treatment decision making in clinical practice.

METHODS

PubMed, Embase, and Google Scholar databases were used to search for literature published in English pertaining to treatment options for erythema related to rosacea. Keywords included "erythematotelangiectatic rosacea," "erythema," "papulopustular rosacea," "brimonidine," "oxymetazoline," "calcineurin inhibitors," "retinoids," "tetracyclines," and "isotretinoin." Treatment types were combined with the keywords "rosacea" and "erythema." Article abstracts were reviewed for relevance to the subject matter, with an emphasis on ETR. Articles included in the review specifically discussed the medical management of rosacea-related erythema, the clinical trials of these treatments, and/or adverse effects of treatment. Articles that did not discuss the medical management of rosacea-related erythema were excluded.

TOPICAL TREATMENTS
Brimonidine

Brimonidine 0.33% topical gel is a topical agent approved for the treatment of persistent facial erythema of rosacea.[11] Brimonidine tartrate is a vasoconstrictive $\alpha2$-adrenergic receptor agonist originally used in the treatment of open-angle glaucoma. Brimonidine tartrate is 1000-fold more selective for the $\alpha2$-adrenergic receptor than the $\alpha1$-adrenergic receptor.[12] It causes direct vasoconstriction of small arteries and veins, leading to constriction of abnormally dilated facial blood vessels in patients with erythema.[11] To a lesser degree, it exerts anti-inflammatory effects.[13] Brimonidine tartrate is a more specific and potent vasoconstrictor of human subcutaneous vessels less than 200 μm in diameter than oxymetazoline, a selective $\alpha1$-adrenergic receptor agonist and partial $\alpha2$-adrenergic receptor agonist. Unlike oxymetazoline, brimonidine tartrate is not active against the 5-hydroxytryptamine 2B receptor, which is related to valvular heart disease after long-term treatment.[13,14]

Multiple studies suggest that brimonidine 0.33% gel is safe and efficacious in the treatment of patients with moderate to severe erythema of rosacea. In these studies, the severity of erythema was measured using the clinician's erythema assessment (CEA) and patient's self-assessment (PSA) scales.[11,15–17] In a dose-response phase 2a study, a single application of brimonidine tartrate gel (0.5% vs 0.18% vs 0.07% vs vehicle) reduced facial erythema in a dose-dependent manner over 12 hours compared with vehicle based on CEA, PSA, and chromameter examinations.[15] Brimonidine tartrate 0.5% gel exhibited the greatest reduction of erythema at all time points over 12 hours, achieving a 2-grade improvement in erythema by both CEA and PSA and by median change in chromameter values ($P<.001$). Reduction in erythema occurred within 30 minutes, with the peak effect lasting 4 to 6 hours after single application. After the peak effect diminished, the erythema did not return to baseline level up to 12 hours after application.[15] A phase 2b dose-response study evaluated brimonidine tartrate gel applied once daily (0.5%, 0.18%, vehicle) and twice daily (0.18%, vehicle) for 4 weeks, followed by a 4-week posttreatment phase.[15] Brimonidine 0.5% gel once daily was the most effective in reducing erythema based on both CEA and PSA. Erythema reduction after 28 days of daily use of brimonidine tartrate 0.5% gel was the same or better than day 1, with results superior to vehicle ($P<.001$). Over the 4-week posttreatment phase, no clinically relevant rebound erythema was noted.[15]

In 2 multicenter, randomized, double-blind, parallel-group, vehicle-controlled phase 3 studies, brimonidine 0.33% gel once daily showed significantly greater efficacy compared with vehicle for all efficacy endpoints, with a faster onset of action and good safety and tolerability profiles.[11] Efficacy, defined as a 2-grade improvement in both CEA and PSA over 12 hours, was significantly greater with brimonidine 0.33% gel in comparison to vehicle. At the end of the study, at least 2-grade reductions in both CEA and PSA were achieved 3 hours after application by 31% and 25% of subjects treated with brimonidine 0.33% gel versus only 11% and 9% of patients treated with vehicle.[11] In a separate open-label, multicenter study, the long-term safety and efficacy of brimonidine 0.33% gel once daily was evaluated over 12 months.[17] Improvement was noted after the first application of brimonidine 0.33% gel with reductions in CEA from 3.1 at baseline to 1.7.

In 2013, the US Food and Drug Administration (FDA) approved brimonidine 0.33% gel for the treatment of persistent facial erythema of rosacea. A meta-analysis in 2015 found that there was high-quality evidence to support the effectiveness of topical brimonidine for rosacea.[7] Long-term studies indicate that adverse events are typically dermatologic in nature and mild or moderate in intensity. The most common adverse effects were flushing (9.1%), worsening of erythema (6.5%), or burning sensation of the skin (3.3%).[17] The occurrence of severe, transient rebound erythema several hours after application has been reported.[18] Persistent erythema in the skin adjacent to the site of brimonidine application has also been reported.[19] Patients should be counseled about these potential adverse effects before therapy. In order to minimize adverse effects of brimonidine treatment, general measures such as patient education, adequate skin care, and optimization of brimonidine application (eg, titration of dose) should be used.[20]

Oxymetazoline

Oxymetazoline, a structural derivative of xylometazoline, is an α-adrenergic receptor agonist used for the treatment of nasal congestion that may be efficacious for facial erythema in rosacea. In 2017, the FDA approved oxymetazoline 1% cream for reducing persistent facial erythema associated with rosacea in adults as a result of 2 randomized trials.[21] Xylometazoline and oxymetazoline are highly selective for the α1-adrenoreceptor and partially selective for the α2-adrenoreceptor.[14,22] These adrenoreceptor agonists are under evaluation for treatment of rosacea erythema because of their role in neurovascular regulation and their ability to reversibly constrict peripheral vasculature.[1,23]

Once-daily topical application of oxymetazoline 0.05% solution or xylometazoline 0.05% solution reduced diffuse facial erythema in patients with ETR that were unresponsive to other topical treatments and oral antibiotics.[22,24] In 3 patients with ETR treated with oxymetazoline 0.05% solution once daily (N = 2) and xylometazoline 0.05% solution once daily (N = 1), reduction in facial erythema was observed within 1 to 3 hours. The reduction in erythema reduction persisted throughout the day and remained effective over 8–17 months.

Two phase 3, open-label clinical trials evaluated the safety and efficacy of oxymetazoline 1.0% cream in patients with persistent erythema associated with rosacea. A total of 885 adults with rosacea applied either oxymetazoline or vehicle once daily for 29 days.[21] More patients in the oxymetazoline groups achieved the primary efficacy endpoint (at least a 2-grade reduction in erythema from baseline on both CEA and PSA at 3, 6, 9, and 12 hours after application) than in the vehicle groups. At the end of the first trial, 12% and 6%

of patients receiving oxymetazoline and vehicle achieved the endpoint 3 hours after application, respectively. In the second trial, this was achieved by 14% and 7% of patients in the oxymetazoline and vehicle groups, respectively. Side effects of oxymetazoline include application site dermatitis, worsening of inflammatory rosacea lesions, pain, pruritus, and erythema.[21]

OFF-LABEL TOPICAL TREATMENTS

Although data are limited, a variety of non-FDA-approved topical agents are available for the treatment of rosacea-related erythema. These agents include topical calcineurin inhibitors (eg, tacrolimus, pimecrolimus), permethrin, crotamiton, ivermectin, and retinoids. Therapeutic benefits have been observed in some cases; however, data are limited to a few studies, and only a relatively small number of patients have been treated with these alternative topical agents. These potential topical treatments require further validation in larger, well-controlled studies.

Calcineurin Inhibitors

Topical calcineurin inhibitors like tacrolimus 0.1% ointment and pimecrolimus 1% cream have mixed results for use in ETR and PPR.[25–28] Calcineurin inhibitors have anti-inflammatory and immunomodulatory effects by selectively targeting T cells and mast cells, preventing the production and release of cytokines and other inflammatory mediators.[29] In contrast to corticosteroids, calcineurin inhibitors do not cause telangiectasias and skin atrophy. Because of the inhibitory effects on pro-inflammatory mediators, topical calcineurin inhibitors are expected to be effective in patients with various forms of rosacea.

In an open-label randomized trial with pimecrolimus 1% cream applied over 4 weeks, there was reduction in rosacea clinical scores at the end of 4 weeks (P<.05).[25] Clinical efficacy was evaluated by the standard rosacea grading system developed by the National Rosacea Society Expert Committee and using photographic documentation and a mexameter. The 26 patients who completed the study experienced significantly reduced rosacea clinical scores from 9.65 ± 1.79 at baseline to 7.27 ± 2.11 at the end of treatment (P<.05). The mexameter-measured erythema index decreased significantly from 418.54 ± 89.56 at baseline to 382.23 ± 80.04 at week 4 (P<.05). The greatest response was observed in the first 2 weeks, whereas symptom improvement plateaued in the following 2 weeks.[25] A single-blind, placebo-controlled, split-face trial evaluated the use of pimecrolimus 1% cream over 4 weeks.[28]

There was significant improvement in the erythema score and total rosacea severity score obtained on the pimecrolimus-applied hemi-face after 2 weeks. In addition, 54.16% of patients reported improved subjective symptoms with pimecrolimus compared with 12.50% for placebo.[28]

An open-label trial of tacrolimus 0.1% ointment in patients with ETR or PPR subtypes was conducted over a period of 12 weeks.[26] Dermatologists evaluated erythema on a scale from 0 (none) to 10 (most severe), number of papulopustules, and overall severity of rosacea on a scale from 0 (none) to 10 (most severe) at baseline and at the end of the treatment. At 12 weeks, there was improvement in erythema scores for both the ETR and the PPR groups: from 6.2 ± 0.6 to 4.6 ± 0.6 ($P<.05$) in the ETR group and 5.3 ± 0.7 to 2.9 ± 0.3 ($P<.05$) in the PPR group. There was no decrease in the number of papulopustular lesions.[26]

In some patients, treatment with topical calcineurin inhibitors has been associated with exacerbation of rosacea. Pimecrolimus and tacrolimus may induce a rosacea-like dermatitis.[5] It has been proposed that the immunosuppressive properties of tacrolimus might facilitate the overgrowth of follicular Demodex folliculorum mites and bacteria in susceptible patients.[30] Because topical calcineurin inhibitors have mixed results in the treatment of rosacea and are sometimes cost-prohibitive, off-label use should be restricted to treatment-resistant scenarios or if there is a concomitant inflammatory disease present.

Permethrin, Crotamiton, Ivermectin

Several topical therapies that target D folliculorum and Demodex brevis mites are being investigated in the treatment of rosacea.[31] These antiparasitic agents include permethrin 5%, crotamiton 10%, and ivermectin 1%. They are primarily used to treat PPR, although some studies suggest they may have some utility in improving rosacea-associated erythema.

Oral ivermectin plus topical permethrin effectively resolved a rosacea-like facial Demodex infestation in an immunocompromised patient.[32] Topical permethrin cream maintained these results, and no recurrence was reported after 1-year follow-up. In another case, a patient with numerous Demodex mites was prescribed a regimen of oral ivermectin followed by topical permethrin. Symptomatic relief occurred within 2 weeks, and weekly topical permethrin was efficacious in maintaining results.[33] A double-blind, placebo-controlled, split-face trial evaluated the use of topical permethrin versus placebo on Demodex density and clinical presentations of rosacea for 12 weeks. Use of permethrin improved both transient and nontransient erythema and decreased Demodex density.[34] In a randomized, double-blind, placebo-controlled trial comparing topical permethrin versus metronidazole 0.75% for the treatment of PPR for 8 weeks, permethrin was more effective than placebo and as effective as metronidazole in reducing both erythema and papules. However, it had no effect on telangiectasias.[35]

Crotamiton is typically used for the treatment of scabies, but has been studied in rosacea. In a retrospective analysis of patients with rosacea-like dermatitis, crotamiton 10% twice daily resulted in a 50% or greater reduction in erythema, dryness, scaling, and roughness in 90.6% of patients.[36] Patients had improvement even when diagnostic testing did not confirm the presence of Demodex mites. Although topical crotamiton 10% or permethrin 5% has been used to reduce the numbers of D folliculorum, they are frequently irritating and are therefore not well tolerated.

Ivermectin is a strong acaricide with efficacy against Demodex. Its anti-inflammatory effects are achieved through decreasing neutrophil phagocytosis and chemotaxis, inhibiting inflammatory cytokines and upregulating the anti-inflammatory cytokine interleukin-10.[37,38] These anti-inflammatory properties have prompted the use of topical ivermectin in several conditions, including rosacea.[39] A phase 3, randomized, investigator-blinded clinical trial compared the efficacy and safety of topical ivermectin 1% versus topical metronidazole 0.75% in subjects with PPR over a 16-week treatment period plus a 36-week extension period.[40] Ivermectin was superior to metronidazole in reducing inflammatory lesions from baseline to week 16 (83% vs 73.7%, respectively). A greater number of patients in the ivermectin group were clear or almost clear based on investigator global assessment. However, erythema was not directly addressed.

TOPICAL RETINOIDS

Topical retinoids repair photo-damaged skin by promoting connective tissue remodeling and downregulation of toll-like receptor 2 expression. The mechanism of action is the basis for retinoid efficacy in decreasing rosacea symptoms.[1] In a randomized, double-blind trial, 22 patients with severe or recalcitrant rosacea were divided into 3 groups to compare low-dose oral isotretinoin, topical tretinoin, and combined use of both isotretinoin and tretinoin for 16 weeks. Each treatment group had improvement in erythema and the number of papules and pustules. Although treatment with oral isotretinoin had a more rapid onset of improvement, there were no differences between groups after 16 weeks.[41] In a randomized, double-blind, placebo-controlled study evaluating the efficacy of tretinoin 0.025% and clindamycin 1.2% combination gel in patients with PPR, treatment with the combination gel improved the telangiectatic component of rosacea, whereas no significant difference in papule or pustule count was noted at 12 weeks. The investigators concluded that the tretinoin-clindamycin gel was better suited for the ETR subtype rather than the PPR subtype.[42]

SYSTEMIC AGENTS

If erythema is extensive or not well controlled with topical medications, oral medications such as tetracyclines or β-blockers may be recommended.[6] Oral treatments may be combined with topical treatments initially. As the clinical features of rosacea improve, discontinuation of the systemic agent with continuation of topical treatments may be attempted. In certain patients, improvement can be maintained by continuation of the topical treatment alone after a course of systemic therapy.[6] However, there are limited data on the use of oral agents in the treatment of ETR compared with PPR.

Tetracyclines

The underlying pathophysiology of rosacea results in inflammation that is responsive to antibiotics and has led to the use of tetracyclines, including doxycycline, minocycline, and tetracycline.[1] The antimicrobial activity of these agents is both dose and concentration dependent, and each has anti-inflammatory activity at lower doses than those required to achieve a bactericidal affect.[43,44] Sub-antimicrobial dosing limits the plasma concentration to a range below the minimum inhibitory concentrations for susceptible bacteria.[45] Sub-antimicrobial dosing allows for fewer side effects and decreased risk of bacterial resistance.[44]

Sub-antimicrobial dosing of doxycycline is thought to reduce inflammation by multiple mechanisms.[46] Cathelicidins are proinflammatory peptides linked to inflammation; they increase vascular growth through downstream signaling. As a result, there is increased vascular proliferation and angiogenesis contributing to the formation of enlarged facial vessels, and chemokine formation leading to persistent diffuse centrofacial erythema.[47,48] Doxycycline decreases the activity of

the kallikrein 5 enzyme, which catalyzes the generation of activated cathelicidins, by indirectly inhibiting the matrix metalloproteinase enzymes responsible for generating activated kallikrein.[46]

Two large, randomized, double-blind, placebo-controlled, phase 3 clinical trials evaluated the anti-inflammatory efficacy of doxycycline.[45] Patients received 40 mg of controlled-released doxycycline or placebo for 16 weeks. In the first trial, the mean reduction from baseline in mean CEA score was significantly greater in the actively treated subject arm than the placebo group ($P = .017$). In the second trial, facial erythema decreased, but there was no difference between the study groups.[5] Although both studies used the CEA scale, neither study assessed the effect of doxycycline in patients with only ETR.

Several studies demonstrate the efficacy of sub-antimicrobial dose doxycycline in the treatment of PPR, both as monotherapy and in combination with topical therapy.[18–22,35–38,43–48] Sub-antimicrobial dose doxycycline reduces papules, pustules, and overall facial erythema.[48,52] In a study evaluating the use of the doxycycline 40 mg in adults with PPR for 12 weeks, approximately 75% of the participants with mild to severe rosacea at baseline were clear or almost clear by week 12. Seventy-five percent of participants had CEA scores reflecting no or mild erythema by the end of the study.[53]

Antihypertensive Medications

Antihypertensive drugs, β-adrenergic antagonists in particular, may be used off label for the treatment of rosacea. β-Adrenergic antagonists block the arterial β2-adrenergic receptor, resulting in vasoconstriction of the cutaneous arterial blood vessels and decreased erythema and flushing in some rosacea patients.[49] The β-adrenergic antagonists, nadolol, propranolol, and carvedilol, suppress flushing reactions, particularly when associated with anxiety.[50] There are only a few reports of β-adrenergic antagonist treatment in patients with rosacea.

In a study comparing the efficacy and safety of propranolol, doxycycline, and combination therapy (propranolol plus doxycycline) in patients with rosacea for 12 weeks, propranolol and the combination group had rapid initial improvement within 4 weeks, but all treatment groups had the same effectiveness at the end of the treatment period. The propranolol group had the largest decrease in flushing score after 12 week, compared with the doxycycline and combination group.[50]

Carvedilol, a nonselective β-adrenergic antagonist, has antioxidant and anti-inflammatory actions that have been investigated for the treatment of rosacea.[49,51] One report evaluated the use of carvedilol in refractory facial flushing and persistent erythema of rosacea.[51] Carvedilol successfully reduced both transient flushing and persistent erythema in a patient with severe refractory symptoms. Within 2 weeks, carvedilol therapy (6.25 mg twice daily for 1 week followed by 6.25 mg 3 times a day) dramatically improved the facial erythema. There were no events of hypotension or bradycardia. The patient's assessment of severity based on a 10-point visual analogue scale was reduced from a score of 10 to a score of 1. The patient was maintained on a regimen of carvedilol, doxycycline, and topical pimecrolimus.[51] In a follow-up study, researchers reported successful treatment with carvedilol in 11 normotensive patients with rosacea.[49] The carvedilol dose was titrated from 3.25 mg 3 times a day to 25 mg per day. Assessments included facial erythema, cheek temperature, patient assessment of severity, and adverse events. All patients experienced significant clinical improvement within 3 weeks, with a mean reduction of 2.2°C in cheek temperature and reported improvement of erythema. Side effects were minimal, with only 1 patient discontinuing treatment because of asymptomatic hypotension.[49] Although this study demonstrated that low-dose carvedilol was effective in treating ETR, further prospective controlled studies of carvedilol therapy for ETR are necessary.

Isotretinoin

Isotretinoin is a synthetic retinoid derived from retinol that is primarily used for the treatment of severe, refractory, inflammatory acne. The efficacy of isotretinoin in rosacea may be related to its anti-inflammatory, antioxidative, antiangiogenic, and antifibrotic properties.[54] Although not approved by the FDA for the treatment of rosacea, oral isotretinoin dose ranges of 0.5 to 1.0 mg/kg daily are an effective treatment for severe PPR.[7] Low-dose isotretinoin (10 mg daily) is effective in treating refractory rosacea with fewer adverse effects.[55] Pustular lesions respond rapidly, but a decline in erythema and telangiectasias has also been observed.[56]

In a study comparing oxytetracycline (250 mg twice daily) and isotretinoin (30 mg daily) for 8 weeks in patients with ETR or PPR, both groups experienced clinical improvement, but the oxytetracycline group had better global assessment scores (reduction of erythema, papules, and pustules).[57] Researchers proposed that isotretinoin's reduction of erythema may have been limited by the xerosis and dermatitis associated with its use. In a study investigating the utility of isotretinoin 20 mg daily in the treatment of rosacea-associated erythema, isotretinoin treatment significantly reduced erythema over a period of 4 weeks as measured by dermatologists' and patients' erythema scores. Further reduction in erythema scores was observed until the fifth month, but these were not statistically significant.[58]

SUMMARY

Rosacea continues to pose a clinical challenge. Transient or persistent erythema is the most common symptom, with considerable unmet needs in the rosacea patient population.[59] There have been few effective treatments for erythema, and patients are often advised to avoid triggers. The welcome addition of topical brimonidine and oxymetazoline provides hope that new therapies may soon be available for reducing rosacea-related erythema.

The paucity of large-scale clinical trials in patients with the ETR subtype makes it difficult to draw firm conclusions regarding treatment. Although certain topical and oral treatments appear to have modest benefit in reducing erythema, there is a need for high-quality, well-designed, and rigorously reported studies for the treatments for rosacea. Future trials should be based on a standardized scale of the participant's assessment of the treatment efficacy; uniform scales that reflect global evaluation, erythema, and assessment of telangiectasias should be used.

DISCLOSURE STATEMENT

A. Cline and S.P. McGregor have nothing to disclose. S.R. Feldman is a speaker for Janssen and Taro. He is a consultant and speaker for Galderma, Stiefel/GlaxoSmithKline, Abbott Labs, and Leo Pharma Inc. S.R. Feldman has received grants from Galderma, Janssen, Abbott Labs, Amgen, Stiefel/GlaxoSmithKline, Celgene, and Anacor. He is a consultant for Amgen, Baxter, Caremark, Gerson Lehrman Group, Guidepoint Global, Hanall Pharmaceutical Co Ltd, Kikaku, Lilly, Merck & Co Inc, Merz Pharmaceuticals, Mylan, Novartis Pharmaceuticals, Pfizer Inc, Qurient, Suncare Research, and Xenoport. He is on an advisory board for Pfizer Inc. S.R. Feldman is the founder and holds stock in Causa Research and holds stock and is majority owner in Medical Quality Enhancement Corporation. He receives Royalties from UpToDate and Xlibris.

REFERENCES

1. Steinhoff M, Buddenkotte J, Aubert J, et al. Clinical, cellular, and molecular aspects in the pathophysiology of rosacea. J Investig Dermatol Symp Proc 2011;15(1):2–11.

2. Del Rosso JQ, Gallo RL, Kircik L, et al. Why is rosacea considered to be an inflammatory disorder? The primary role, clinical relevance, and therapeutic correlations of abnormal innate immune response in rosacea-prone skin. J Drugs Dermatol 2012;11(6): 694–700.

3. Wilkin J, Dahl M, Detmar M, et al. Standard grading system for rosacea: report of the National Rosacea Society Expert Committee on the classification and staging of rosacea. J Am Acad Dermatol 2004; 50(6):907–12.

4. Hengge UR, Ruzicka T, Schwartz RA, et al. Adverse effects of topical glucocorticosteroids. J Am Acad Dermatol 2006;54(1):1–15 [quiz: 16–8].

5. Teraki Y, Hitomi K, Sato Y, et al. Tacrolimus-induced rosacea-like dermatitis: a clinical analysis of 16 cases associated with tacrolimus ointment application. Dermatology 2012;224(4):309–14.

6. Elewski BE, Draelos Z, Dreno B, et al. Rosacea—global diversity and optimized outcome: proposed international consensus from the Rosacea International Expert Group. J Eur Acad Dermatol Venereol 2011;25(2):188–200.

7. van Zuuren EJ, Fedorowicz Z, Carter B, et al. Interventions for rosacea. Cochrane Database Syst Rev 2015;(4):CD003262.

8. Thiboutot D, Thieroff-Ekerdt R, Graupe K. Efficacy and safety of azelaic acid (15%) gel as a new treatment for papulopustular rosacea: results from two vehicle-controlled, randomized phase III studies. J Am Acad Dermatol 2003;48(6):836–45.

9. Maddin S. A comparison of topical azelaic acid 20% cream and topical metronidazole 0.75% cream in the treatment of patients with papulopustular rosacea. J Am Acad Dermatol 1999;40(6 Pt 1):961–5.

10. Breneman D, Savin R, VandePol C, et al. Double-blind, vehicle-controlled clinical trial of once-daily benzoyl peroxide/clindamycin topical gel in the treatment of patients with moderate to severe rosacea. Int J Dermatol 2004;43(5):381–7.

11. Fowler J Jr, Jackson M, Moore A, et al. Efficacy and safety of once-daily topical brimonidine tartrate gel 0.5% for the treatment of moderate to severe facial erythema of rosacea: results of two randomized, double-blind, and vehicle-controlled pivotal studies. J Drugs Dermatol 2013;12(6):650–6.

12. Tong LX, Moore AY. Brimonidine tartrate for the treatment of facial flushing and erythema in rosacea. Expert Rev Clin Pharmacol 2014;7(5):567–77.

13. Piwnica D, Rosignoli C, de Menonville ST, et al. Vasoconstriction and anti-inflammatory properties of the selective alpha-adrenergic receptor agonist brimonidine. J Dermatol Sci 2014;75(1):49–54.

14. Huang XP, Setola V, Yadav PN, et al. Parallel functional activity profiling reveals valvulopathogens are potent 5-hydroxytryptamine(2B) receptor agonists: implications for drug safety assessment. Mol Pharmacol 2009;76(4):710–22.

15. Fowler J, Jarratt M, Moore A, et al. Once-daily topical brimonidine tartrate gel 0.5% is a novel treatment for moderate to severe facial erythema of rosacea: results of two multicentre, randomized and vehicle-controlled studies. Br J Dermatol 2012; 166(3):633–41.

16. Jackson JM, Fowler J, Moore A, et al. Improvement in facial erythema within 30 minutes of initial application of brimonidine tartrate in patients with rosacea. J Drugs Dermatol 2014;13(6):699–704.

17. Moore A, Kempers S, Murakawa G, et al. Long-term safety and efficacy of once-daily topical brimonidine tartrate gel 0.5% for the treatment of moderate to severe facial erythema of rosacea: results of a 1-year open-label study. J Drugs Dermatol 2014;13(1): 56–61.

18. Routt ET, Levitt JO. Rebound erythema and burning sensation from a new topical brimonidine tartrate gel 0.33%. J Am Acad Dermatol 2014; 70(2):e37–8.

19. Gillihan R, Nguyen T, Fischer R, et al. Erythema in skin adjacent to area of long-term brimonidine treatment for rosacea: a novel adverse reaction. JAMA Dermatol 2015;151(10):1136–7.

20. Tanghetti EA, Jackson JM, Belasco KT, et al. Optimizing the use of topical brimonidine in rosacea management: panel recommendations. J Drugs Dermatol 2015;14(1):33–40.

21. Allergan announces FDA approval of RHOFADE™ (oxymetazoline hydrochloride) cream, 1% for the topical treatment of persistent facial erythema associated with rosacea in adults. Rhofade [package insert]. Irvine (CA): Allergan; 2017.

22. Shanler SD, Ondo AL. Successful treatment of the erythema and flushing of rosacea using a topically applied selective alpha1-adrenergic receptor agonist, oxymetazoline. Arch Dermatol 2007; 143(11):1369–71.

23. Schwab VD, Sulk M, Seeliger S, et al. Neurovascular and neuroimmune aspects in the pathophysiology of rosacea. J Investig Dermatol Symp Proc 2011;15(1): 53–62.

24. Kim JH, Oh YS, Ji JH, et al. Rosacea (erythematotelangiectatic type) effectively improved by topical xylometazoline. J Dermatol 2011;38(5):510–3.

25. Kim M-B, Kim G-W, Park H-J, et al. Pimecrolimus 1% cream for the treatment of rosacea. J Dermatol 2011;38(12):1135–9.

26. Bamford JT, Elliott BA, Haller IV. Tacrolimus effect on rosacea. J Am Acad Dermatol 2004;50(1):107–8.

27. Weissenbacher S, Merkl J, Hildebrandt B, et al. Pimecrolimus cream 1% for papulopustular rosacea: a randomized vehicle-controlled double-blind trial. Br J Dermatol 2007;156(4):728–32.

28. Karabulut AA, Serel BI, Eksioglu HM. A randomized, single-blind, placebo-controlled, split-face study with pimecrolimus cream 1% for papulopustular rosacea. J Eur Acad Dermatol Venereol 2008;22(6): 729–34.

29. Gupta AK, Chow M. Pimecrolimus: a review. J Eur Acad Dermatol Venereol 2003;17(5):493–503.

30. Fujiwara S, Okubo Y, Irisawa R, et al. Rosaceiform dermatitis associated with topical tacrolimus treatment. J Am Acad Dermatol 2010;62(6): 1050–2.

31. Layton A, Thiboutot D. Emerging therapies in rosacea. J Am Acad Dermatol 2013;69(6 Suppl 1): S57–65.

32. Aquilina C, Viraben R, Sire S. Ivermectin-responsive demodex infestation during human immunodeficiency virus infection. Dermatology 2002;205(4): 394–7.

33. Forstinger C, Kittler H, Binder M. Treatment of rosacea-like demodicidosis with oral ivermectin and topical permethrin cream. J Am Acad Dermatol 1999;41(5):775–7.

34. Raoufinejad K, Mansouri P, Rajabi M, et al. Efficacy and safety of permethrin 5% topical gel vs. placebo for rosacea: a double-blind randomized controlled clinical trial. J Eur Acad Dermatol Venereol 2016; 30(12):2105–17.

35. Kocak M, Yagli S, Vahapoglu G, et al. Permethrin 5% cream versus metronidazole 0.75% gel for the treatment of papulopustular rosacea. A randomized double-blind placebo-controlled study. Dermatology 2002;205(3):265–70.

36. Bikowski JB, Del Rosso JQ. Demodex dermatitis: a retrospective analysis of clinical diagnosis and successful treatment with topical crotamiton. J Clin Aesthet Dermatol 2009;2(1):20–5.

37. Stein L, Kircik L, Fowler J, et al. Efficacy and safety of ivermectin 1% cream in treatment of papulopustular rosacea: results of two randomized, double-blind, vehicle-controlled pivotal studies. J Drugs Dermatol 2014;13(3):316–23.

38. Abokwidir M, Fleischer AB. An emerging treatment: topical ivermectin for papulopustular rosacea. J Dermatolog Treat 2015;26(4):379–80.

39. Clyti E, Nacher M, Sainte-Marie D, et al. Ivermectin treatment of three cases of demodecidosis during human immunodeficiency virus infection. Int J Dermatol 2006;45(9):1066–8.

40. Taieb A, Ortonne JP, Ruzicka T, et al. Superiority of ivermectin 1% cream over metronidazole 0.75% cream in treating inflammatory lesions of rosacea: a randomized, investigator-blinded trial. Br J Dermatol 2015;172(4):1103–10.

41. Ertl GA, Levine N, Kligman AM. A comparison of the efficacy of topical tretinoin and low-dose oral isotretinoin in rosacea. Arch Dermatol 1994;130(3): 319–24.

42. Chang AL, Alora-Palli M, Lima XT, et al. A randomized, double-blind, placebo-controlled, pilot study to assess the efficacy and safety of clindamycin 1.2% and tretinoin 0.025% combination gel for the treatment of acne rosacea over 12 weeks. J Drugs Dermatol 2012;11(3):333–9.

43. Sneddon IB. A clinical trial of tetracycline in rosacea. Br J Dermatol 1966;78(12):649–52.

44. Bikowski JB. Subantimicrobial dose doxycycline for acne and rosacea. Skinmed 2003;2(4):234–45.

45. Del Rosso JQ, Webster GF, Jackson M, et al. Two randomized phase III clinical trials evaluating anti-inflammatory dose doxycycline (40-mg doxycycline, USP capsules) administered once daily for treatment of rosacea. J Am Acad Dermatol 2007;56(5): 791–802.

46. Kanada KN, Nakatsuji T, Gallo RL. Doxycycline indirectly inhibits proteolytic activation of tryptic kallikrein-related peptidases and activation of cathelicidin. J Invest Dermatol 2012;132(5):1435–42.

47. Yamasaki K, Gallo RL. Rosacea as a disease of cathelicidins and skin innate immunity. J Investig Dermatol Symp Proc 2011;15(1):12–5.

48. Del Rosso JQ. Advances in understanding and managing rosacea: part 1: connecting the dots between pathophysiological mechanisms and common clinical features of rosacea with emphasis on vascular changes and facial erythema. J Clin Aesthet Dermatol 2012;5(3):16–25.

49. Hsu CC, Lee JY. Pronounced facial flushing and persistent erythema of rosacea effectively treated by carvedilol, a nonselective beta-adrenergic blocker. J Am Acad Dermatol 2012;67:491–3.

50. Park JM, Mun JH, Song M, et al. Propranolol, doxycycline and combination therapy for the treatment of rosacea. J Dermatol 2015;42(1):64–9.

51. Hsu CC, Lee JY. Carvedilol for the treatment of refractory facial flushing and persistent erythema of rosacea. Arch Dermatol 2011;147(11):1258–60.

52. van Zuuren EJ, Kramer S, Carter B, et al. Interventions for rosacea. Cochrane Database Syst Rev 2011;(3):CD003262.

53. Webster GF. An open-label, community-based, 12-week assessment of the effectiveness and safety of monotherapy with doxycycline 40 mg (30-mg immediate-release and 10-mg delayed-release beads). Cutis 2010;86(5 Suppl):7–15.

54. Rallis E, Korfitis C. Isotretinoin for the treatment of granulomatous rosacea: case report and review of the literature. J Cutan Med Surg 2012;16(6):438–41.

55. Park H, Del Rosso JQ. Use of oral isotretinoin in the management of rosacea. J Clin Aesthet Dermatol 2011;4(9):54–61.

56. Erdogan FG, Yurtsever P, Aksoy D, et al. Efficacy of low-dose isotretinoin in patients with treatment-resistant rosacea. Arch Dermatol 1998;134(7):884–5.

57. Irvine C, Kumar P, Marks R. Isotretinoin in the treatment of rosacea and rhinophyma. London: 1988.

58. Uslu M, Savk E, Karaman G, et al. Rosacea treatment with intermediate-dose isotretinoin: follow-up with erythema and sebum measurements. Acta Derm Venereol 2012;92(1):73–7.

59. Del Rosso JQ. Advances in understanding and managing rosacea: part 2: the central role, evaluation, and medical management of diffuse and persistent facial erythema of rosacea. J Clin Aesthet Dermatol 2012;5(3):26–36.

Revisiting Rosacea Criteria
Where Have We Been, Where Are We Going, and How Will We Get There?

Mohammed D. Saleem, MD, MPH

KEYWORDS

- Evidence-based • Criteria • Assessment • Management

KEY POINTS

- A valid case definition of rosacea is critical for the appropriate interpretation and external validity of research studies.
- Current criteria for rosacea are based on expert opinion.
- Incorporating techniques from other specialties can improve the reliability and validity of rosacea criteria and help advance understanding of rosacea in the future.

INTRODUCTION

Rosacea, first noted in the fourteenth century,[1] is one of the most common and misunderstood dermatologic conditions.[2] The depiction of rosacea, throughout history, altered with advancing imaging technologies.[3] Today, rosacea is defined by recognizable morphologic features but without any single laboratory, pathologic, or radiologic feature serving as a pathognomonic gold standard.[4–6] As a result, rosacea criteria are intended to provide a consensus standard to ascertain cases in a consistent manner across clinical and epidemiologic studies. A valid case definition of rosacea is fundamentally critical for interpretation and external validity of epidemiologic and clinical studies. Nonvalid criteria unnecessarily incorporate subjects without disease into clinical studies.[7] Unfortunately, the definition of rosacea and its subgroups has been driven more by impressions and opinions than by evidence. As a result, empiric data underpinning the reliability and validity of rosacea criteria are lacking, which has hindered understanding of rosacea and contributed to conflicting scientific results.[5,8–26]

CURRENT ROSACEA CRITERIA

In 2002, a National Rosacea Society consensus (NRSC) committee developed provisional diagnostic and classification criteria based on phenotypic features and scientific knowledge.[27] The purpose was to establish standard terminology that would improve communication globally, allow study comparisons, and advance epidemiologic, pathophysiologic, and clinical understanding of rosacea. According to the diagnostic criteria, the presence of 1 or more primary features (flushing, erythema, papules and pustules, and telangiectasia) in a centrofacial distribution is indicative of rosacea.[27] Multiple concerns or questions need to be addressed because lack of specificity can be harmful.[28] For instance, is the sole presence of facial flushing in women diagnostic? If so, 88% of women between 40 years and 65 years of age have rosacea.[29] Are multiple inflammatory papules distributed over the cheeks rosacea? Can rosacea be diagnosed in a patient with facial erythema after a weekend at the beach? Is the presence of centrofacial telangiectasias associated with extrinsic aging adequate to establishing a diagnosis of rosacea? Recently, the global

Disclosure Statement: The author has nothing to disclose.
University of Florida College of Medicine, PO Box 100277, Gainesville, Fl 32610-0277, USA
E-mail address: msaleem@g.clemson.edu

Dermatol Clin 36 (2018) 161–165
https://doi.org/10.1016/j.det.2017.11.011

ROSacea Consensus panel re-evaluated and recommended updated criteria for diagnosis, classification, and assessment of rosacea.[30] Both the National Rosacea Society consensus and ROSacea Consensus criteria were synthesized from expert opinion. Neither addresses validity or reliability nor have they been tested in subsequent studies.

Diagnostic or classification criteria for disease diagnosis that are based solely on expert opinion are tentative, at best. Expert opinion is susceptible to various biases; frequently, their precision and accuracy are decreased when they are applied to a general clinical setting. For example, the Jones criteria establish a set of features diagnostic of rheumatic fever based on expert opinion.[31] In certain populations, the Jones criteria had altered validity, resulting in rheumatic fever missed with subsequent devastating health consequences.[32] Importantly, the weaknesses were identified and the American Heart Association revised the criteria to reflect current epidemiologic trends and advancing scientific knowledge. The purpose of revisiting previous criteria is not to criticize but to incorporate novel knowledge and current literature to improve reliability and validity of criteria.[33]

PURPOSE AND OBJECTIVES OF ROSACEA CRITERIA

Synthesizing rosacea criteria requires that an objective be predefined. Frequently, rosacea diagnostic and classification criteria are intertwined in clinical and epidemiologic interpretations, which have limited scientific progression and masked potential insight into advancing our understanding of rosacea.[5] Diagnostic and classification criteria are modeled differently and should be distinguished. A diagnosis is the end outcome of a process that incorporates a physician's skill, knowledge, and intuition that aims to confirm or deny the presence of a health condition. The purpose is to guide patient care and predict prognosis. The process is complex and incorporates individual weights for variables that differ between clinicians, settings, and patients.[34] Even the most basic features of rosacea are disagreed on. For instance, approximately 30%, from an expert panel, disagree that flushing is a major feature of rosacea.[30] In the absence of a gold standard, rarely is a single diagnostic criterion adequate because of different disease prevalence and presentations among different populations; for these reasons, the American College of Rheumatology no longer endorses diagnostic criteria.[35] In contrast, classification criteria are intended to define a cohort of subjects with a shared set of homogenous features for clinical research.[36] They

should standardize the definition of rosacea and its subtypes across various populations. As a result, the external validity of rosacea studies is protected by minimizing identification bias; in other words, the sample is a true representation of the disease, ensuring the same disease entity is studied consistently.

Rosacea criteria validity, which can be measured by sensitivity and specificity, is defined by its ability to distinguish rosacea from other conditions. Most importantly, the criteria should focus on maximizing construct validity, that is, the criteria correlate with clinical construct (convergent validity) and diverge from other conditions (divergent validity).[37] In this paradigm, optimal evaluation and diagnosis of rosacea incorporate current scientific knowledge (increasing diagnostic sensitivity) and exclude diseases with similar phenotypic features (increasing diagnostic specificity).[38] Diagnostic disagreements, beyond training and experience, arise primarily from inadequate nosology; often due to nonspecific criteria.[39]

SYNTHESIZING VALID CRITERIA FOR ROSACEA

Using evidence and historical lessons from other specialties can provide a framework for developing valid rosacea criteria. Diagnostic and classification criteria are used widely in psychiatry and rheumatology due to the lack of a single gold standard test. The *Diagnostic and Statistical Manual* (*DSM*) was developed in response to multiple landmark studies that demonstrated frequent diagnostic disagreement.[40] Initially, the first edition of the *DSM* and the *DSM* (Second Edition) had low reliability; subsequent revisions improved its reliability and diagnostic agreement among clinicians.[41,42] Similarly, classification criteria in rheumatic disease have consistently been revised to reflect current literature. Well-developed criteria improve clinical decision making and individual care.[43] An approach using a well-defined framework described by the American College of Rheumatology and incorporating evidence-based literature that might produce well-developed and validated criteria for rosacea is outlined.[35]

Synthesizing rosacea classification criteria begins with a formal group consensus method, designed to organize subjective judgements in conjunction with available objective evidence. Universal agreement is not expected; rather, a predefined consensus should identify a central tendency and quantify the level of agreement.[44,45] Panel selection should comprise a heterogeneous group of enthusiastic expert participants that understand the demand and responsibilities required.[44] A literature review should be performed and evidence-based literature should be shared with participants. Scientific literature is influential in the decision-making process and improves the overall quality of the criteria.[46–49] Multiple major formal consensus methods exist, including the Delphi method, nominal group process, National Institutes of Health consensus development, and Glaser's state-of-the-art approach.[45] The Delphi method, widely used for diagnostic and classification criteria, followed by the nominal group process allows a large number of participants and international collaboration that produces criteria sets with a high likelihood of being widely accepted and used.[35,50,51] The Delphi method is a multistage process developed to reduce dominant opinion or pressure to conform to majority opinion by anonymization and controlled feedback.[44,52] Regardless of the technique used, all are accompanied by its own set of limitations.

The list of inclusion and exclusion criteria is applied to an adequate number of cases and controls; the criteria set that best differentiates rosacea (greatest validity, sensitivity, and specificity) from controls is selected.[53] To prevent identification bias, case and control vignettes should be selected prior to the process and by clinicians who are not involved in the criteria development process. Cases should represent the spectrum of rosacea severity and selected from a variety of geographic regions and clinical settings. To be clinically useful and valid, which means the criteria can distinguish rosacea from other conditions, controls should comprise conditions that rosacea must be differentiated from, such as acne, hot flushes, folliculitis, photoaging, and so forth.[37] The final criteria selected should be validated using a large sample that differs from the subjects used to develop the original criteria.[35,53,54]

The process is time consuming and demanding, emphasizing the importance of recruiting enthusiastic experts, but is ultimately rewarding. For example, preliminary criteria for acute gout began with 235 criteria elements, 178 cases of gout, and more than 500 controls collected from 38 centers across the United States. Control vignettes were collected from patients with pseudogout, rheumatoid arthritis, and septic arthritis. Regression analysis narrowed the inclusion elements to 13 and identified criteria that were highly sensitive and specific.[55]

SUMMARY

A valid classification criteria for rosacea is fundamentally essential for clear communication among researchers and health care providers. Maximizing reliability and validity of rosacea criteria requires that it reflect current literature. Reassessing rosacea criteria may be beneficial and warranted to improving case ascertainment; previously neglected, divergent validity should also be considered.

ACKNOWLEDGMENTS

M.D. Saleem thanks Dr Jonathan Wilkin for taking the time to review the article and providing valuable suggestions.

REFERENCES

1. Drake L. Now Widely Recognized, Rosacea Was First Noted in 14th Century. National Rosacea Society. 1996. Available at: https://www.rosacea.org/rr/1996/winter/article_1.php. Accessed November 22, 2017.
2. Olazagasti J, Lynch P, Fazel N. The great mimickers of rosacea. Cutis 2014;94(1):39–45.
3. Cribier B. Medical history of the representation of rosacea in the 19th century. J Am Acad Dermatol 2013;69:S2–14.
4. Fonseca GP, Brenner FM, Muller Cde S, et al. Nailfold capillaroscopy as a diagnostic and prognostic method in rosacea. An Bras Dermatol 2011;86:87–90.
5. Crawford GH, Pelle MT, James WD. Rosacea: I. Etiology, pathogenesis, and subtype classification. J Am Acad Dermatol 2004;51:327–41.
6. Powell FC. The histopathology of rosacea: "where"s the beef?'. Dermatology 2004;209:173–4.
7. Dalbeth N, Fransen J, Jansen TL, et al. New classification criteria for gout: a framework for progress. Rheumatology 2013;52:1748–53.
8. Schaefer I, Rustenbach SJ, Zimmer L, et al. Prevalence of skin diseases in a cohort of 48,665 employees in Germany. Dermatology 2008;217:169–72.
9. Abram K, Silm H, Oona M. Prevalence of rosacea in an estonian working population using a standard classification. Acta Derm Venereol 2010;90:269–73.
10. Spoendlin J, Voegel JJ, Jick SS, et al. A study on the epidemiology of rosacea in the U.K. Br J Dermatol 2012;167:598–605.
11. Lazaridou E, Apalla Z, Sotiraki S, et al. Clinical and laboratory study of rosacea in northern Greece. J Eur Acad Dermatol Venereol 2010;24:410–4.
12. Berg M, Lidén S. An epidemiological study of rosacea. Acta Derm Venereol 1989;69:419–23.
13. Kyriakis KP, Palamaras I, Terzoudi S, et al. Epidemiologic aspects of rosacea. J Am Acad Dermatol 2005;53:918–9.

14. Powell FC. Clinical practice. Rosacea. N Engl J Med 2005;352:793–803.

15. Kligman AM. An experimental critique on the state of knowledge of rosacea. J Cosmet Dermatol 2006; 5(1):77–80.

16. Moustafa F, Hopkinson D, Huang KE, et al. Prevalence of rosacea in community settings. J Cutan Med Surg 2015;19:149–52.

17. Kucukunal A, Altunay I, Arici JE, et al. Is the effect of smoking on rosacea still somewhat of a mystery? Cutan Ocul Toxicol 2015;35:1–5.

18. Quarterman MJ, Johnson DW, Abele DC, et al. Ocular rosacea. Signs, symptoms, and tear studies before and after treatment with doxycycline. Arch Dermatol 1997;133:49–54.

19. Ghanem VC, Mehra N, Wong S, et al. The prevalence of ocular signs in acne rosacea: comparing patients from ophthalmology and dermatology clinics. Cornea 2003;22:230–3.

20. Browning DJ, Rosenwasser G, Lugo M. Ocular rosacea in blacks. Am J Ophthalmol 1986;101: 441–4.

21. Rosen T, Stone MS. Acne rosacea in blacks. J Am Acad Dermatol 1987;17:70–3.

22. Alexis AF. Rosacea in patients with skin of color: uncommon but not rare. Cutis 2010;86(2):60–2.

23. Tidman MJ. Improving the management of rosacea in primary care. Practitioner 2014;258:27–30, 3.

24. Tanzi EL, Weinberg JM. The ocular manifestations of rosacea. Cutis 2001;68:112–4.

25. Vieira ACC, Höfling-Lima AL, Mannis MJ. Ocular rosacea–a review. Arq Bras Oftalmol 2012;75: 363–9.

26. Vieira AC, Mannis MJ. Ocular rosacea: common and commonly missed. J Am Acad Dermatol 2013;69: S36–41.

27. Wilkin J, Dahl M, Detmar M, et al. Standard classification of rosacea: report of the national rosacea society expert committee on the classification and staging of rosacea. J Am Acad Dermatol 2002;46: 584–7.

28. Shekelle PG, Kravitz RL, Beart J, et al. Are nonspecific practice guidelines potentially harmful? A randomized comparison of the effect of nonspecific versus specific guidelines on physician decision making. Health Serv Res 2000;34:1429–48.

29. Williams RE, Kalilani L, DiBenedetti DB, et al. Frequency and severity of vasomotor symptoms among peri- and postmenopausal women in the United States. Climacteric 2008;11:32–43.

30. Tan J, Almeida LMC, Bewley A, et al. Updating the diagnosis, classification and assessment of rosacea: recommendations from the global ROSacea COnsensus (ROSCO) panel. Br J Dermatol 2017; 176(2):431–8.

31. Jones T. The diagnosis of rheumatic fever. J Am Med Assoc 1944;126:481.

32. Hajar R. Rheumatic fever and rheumatic heart disease a historical perspective. Heart Views 2016;17: 120–6.

33. Johnson SR, Fransen J, Khanna D, et al. Validation of potential classification criteria for systemic sclerosis. Arthritis Care Res (hoboken) 2012;64: 358–67.

34. Taylor WJ, Fransen J. Distinctions between diagnostic and classification criteria: comment on the article by Aggarwal et al. Arthritis Care Res (hoboken) 2016;68:149–50.

35. Singh JA, Solomon DH, Dougados M, et al. Development of classification and response criteria for rheumatic diseases. Arthritis Rheum 2006;55:348–52.

36. Yazici H. Diagnostic versus classification criteria - a continuum. Bull NYU Hosp Jt Dis 2009;67:206–8.

37. Felson DT, Anderson JJ. Methodological and statistical approaches to criteria development in rheumatic diseases. Baillieres Clin Rheumatol 1995;9: 253–66.

38. Tan J, Steinhoff M, Berg M, et al. Shortcomings in rosacea diagnosis and classification. Br J Dermatol 2017;176:197–9.

39. Ward C, Beck AT, Mendelson M, et al. The psychiatric nomenclature. Reasons for diagnostic disagreement. Arch Gen Psychiatry 1962;7:198–205.

40. Grove WM, Andreasen NC, McDonald-Scott P, et al. Reliability studies of psychiatric diagnosis. Theory and practice. Arch Gen Psychiatry 1981;38:408–13.

41. Spitzer RL, Forman JB, Nee J. DSM-III field trials: I. Initial interrater diagnostic reliability. Am J Psychiatry 1979;136:815–7.

42. Spitzer RL, Endicott J, Williams JB. Research diagnostic criteria. Arch Gen Psychiatry 1979;36: 1381–3.

43. Lugtenberg M, Burgers JS, Westert GP. Effects of evidence-based clinical practice guidelines on quality of care: a systematic review. Qual Saf Heal Care 2009;18:385–92.

44. Nair R, Aggarwal R, Khanna D. Methods of formal consensus in classification/diagnostic criteria and guideline development. Semin Arthritis Rheum 2011;41:95–105.

45. Fink A, Kosecoff J, Chassin M, et al. Consensus methods: characteristics and guidelines for use. Am J Public Health 1984;74:979–83.

46. Cruse H, Winiarek M, Marshburn J, et al. Quality and methods of developing practice guidelines. BMC Health Serv Res 2002;2:1.

47. Vinokur A, Burnstein E, Sechrest L, et al. Group decision making by experts: field study of panels evaluating medical technologies. J Pers Soc Psychol 1985;49:70–84.

48. Jacoby I. Evidence and consensus. JAMA 1988; 259:3039.

49. Jones J, Hunter D. Consensus methods for medical and health services research. BMJ 1995;311:376–80.

50. Jamieson M, Griffiths R, Jayasuriya R. Developing outcomes for community nursing: the Nominal Group Technique. Aust J Adv Nurs 1998;16(1):14–9.

51. Taylor WJ. Preliminary identification of core domains for outcome studies in psoriatic arthritis using delphi methods. Ann Rheum Dis 2005;64(Suppl 2): ii110-2.

52. Hsu C-C, Sandford BA. The Delphi Technique: Making Sense of Consensus. Practical Assessment Research & Evaluation. 2007. http://pareonline.net/ getvn.asp?v=12&n=10. Accessed November 22, 2017.

53. Bloch DA, Moses LE, Michel BA. Statistical approaches to classification. Methods for developing classification and other criteria rules. Arthritis Rheum 1990;33:1137–44.

54. Astion ML, Bloch DA, Wener MH. Neural networks as expert systems in rheumatic disease diagnosis: artificial intelligence or intelligent artifice? J Rheumatol 1993;20:1465–8.

55. Wallace SL, Robinson H, Masi AT, et al. Preliminary criteria for the classification of the acute arthritis of primary gout. Arthritis Rheum 1977; 20:895–900.

Patient Costs Associated with Rosacea

Jackson G. Turbeville, BS[a], Hossein Alinia, MD[a], Sara Moradi Tuchayi, MD, MPH[a], Naeim Bahrami, PhD[a,b], Leah A. Cardwell, MD[a,*], Olabola Awosika, MD, MS[c], Irma Richardson, MHA[a], Karen E. Huang, MS[a], Steven R. Feldman, MD, PhD[a,d,e]

KEYWORDS

- Health care cost • Rosacea • Severity • Self-assessment • Papulopustular
- Erythematotelangiectatic

KEY POINTS

- The recalcitrance of rosacea to many treatment options may prompt patients to spend exorbitant amounts of money on unsubstantiated treatment regimens in an effort to achieve relief.
- There was a significant relationship between the disease severity and the amount of monthly expenses on rosacea treatments ($P = .013$). The highest mean amount spent was in severity levels 6 and 7.
- There was a significant relationship between disease severity and household income ($P<.0001$); patients with higher disease severity levels had lower household incomes.
- Familiarization of evidence-based clinical recommendations and consensus guidelines may equip physicians to educate patients about the most efficacious and cost-effective treatment options.

INTRODUCTION

Rosacea is common and bothersome. It impacts many dimensions of quality of life. There are also many treatment options, some more costly than others. The financial impact—in particular the cost of treatment—has not been well characterized. The authors used a validated self-assessment tool to document severity of rosacea and inquire about spending related to rosacea treatment. They examine the relationship between disease severity and treatment cost across several demographic and socioeconomic strata.

METHODS

Study participants were adult patients from the Wake Forest Baptist Medical Center dermatology clinic from 2011 to 2014 who had received a diagnosis of rosacea (*International Classification of Diseases, Ninth Revision*: 695.3) from a Wake Forest dermatologist. Before initiation, the study was approved by the Institutional Review Board. Data collection occurred from October 2014 through February 2015. A total of 478 patients met criteria for participation in the study. These individuals were identified from the Wake Forest Baptist Hospital

Disclosure: See last page of article.

[a] Department of Dermatology, Center for Dermatology Research, Wake Forest School of Medicine, Medical Center Boulevard, Winston-Salem, NC 27157-1071, USA; [b] Department of Biomedical Engineering, Virginia Polytechnic Institute and State University, Wake Forest University, Medical Center Boulevard, Winston-Salem, NC 27157-1071, USA; [c] Department of Dermatology, The George Washington Medical Faculty Associates, 2150 Pennsylvania Avenue Northwest, 2B-427, Washington, DC 20037, USA; [d] Department of Pathology, Wake Forest School of Medicine, Medical Center Boulevard, Winston-Salem, NC 27157-1071, USA; [e] Department of Public Health Sciences, Wake Forest School of Medicine, Medical Center Boulevard, Winston-Salem, NC 27157-1071, USA

* Corresponding author. Department of Dermatology, Wake Forest School of Medicine, Medical Center Boulevard, Winston-Salem, NC 27157-1071.

E-mail address: lcardwell06@gmail.com

Dermatol Clin 36 (2018) 167–170
https://doi.org/10.1016/j.det.2017.11.012

Transitional Data Warehouse and the electronic medical record. Since rosacea is not typically diagnosed in children and the data measures are not validated in children, this demographic group was excluded from participation.

A total of 165 patients were contacted, via telephone, to complete the survey study in person. Forty-six patients completed the self-assessment tool and survey study in person. A total of 432 potential subjects were mailed a pre-survey recruitment letter notifying them that they would be receiving a survey in the mail unless they contacted the authors to decline participation; study team e-mail and phone number were provided in letter. Twenty patients declined to participate. Surveys were mailed to the remaining 412 individuals.

Of the mailed surveys, 16 were returned because of incorrect address. A total of 195 surveys (149 through mail and 46 in person) were completed and analyzed. All survey responders completed a validated self-assessment tool (**Fig. 1**). Using the self-assessment tool, patients selected images corresponding to the severity of their symptoms; categories included erythema, papulopustular lesions, ocular symptoms, and nasal involvement. Scores on the self-assessment ranged from 2 (least severe) to 8 (most severe). Subjects also answered questions pertaining to estimated out-of-pocket treatment expenses. Subjects participating in this study received compensation for travel expenses and time.

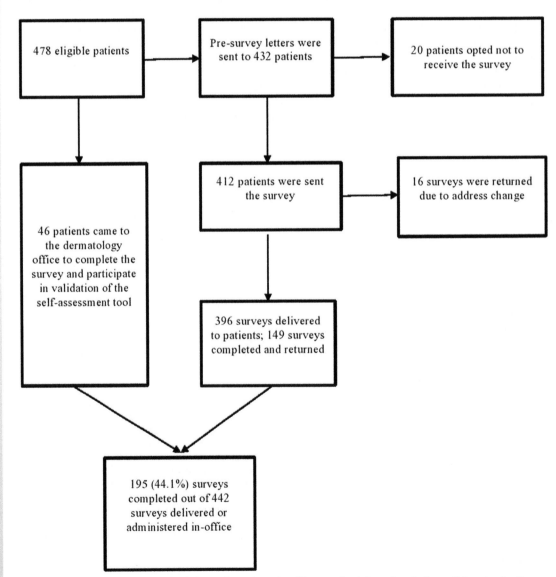

Fig. 1. Participant selection methodology. Flow chart detailing methodology for study participant selection.

Descriptive statistics were used to report results. To study the relationship between treatment expenses, household incomes, and gender, the patients were grouped by disease severity. A Tukey-Kramer Honest Significant Difference test was used to compare all possible combinations of means from groups of severity and expenditures per month. A linear regression analysis was performed to evaluate the correlation between household income and expenditure amount per month on treatments. Comparisons of continuous variables were achieved using the *t* test or analysis of variance, whereas proportions between groups were compared using a χ^2 test.

RESULTS

Nonresponders Versus Responders

A total of 263 patients (44.1%) were nonresponders, and the 16 patients with an incorrect address are included in this group. Nonresponders were 62.4% (n = 169) women, which is comparable to the proportion in responders. Of responders, the sample consisted of more women (n = 155; 81.2%) than men (n = 36; 18.8%).

Expenses (Out of Pocket and Insurance)

Total expenses (including out of pocket and insurance costs) were examined in the whole cohort. Patient groups were separated based on reported rosacea severity. There was a significant relationship between the disease severity and the amount of monthly expenses on rosacea treatments (*P* = .013). The highest mean amount spent was in severity levels 6 and 7 (**Fig. 2**).

Expenses (Out of Pocket)

Monthly out-of-pocket costs were examined in the whole cohort. Patient groups were separated

based on reported rosacea severity. Patients in severity level 4 and 6 were spending significantly more money out of pocket per month than patients in level 2 (*P* = .0216 and *P* = .0136, respectively) (**Fig. 3**).

Alternative Medicines

The data were examined for changes in disease status and the amount of money spent per month on alternative treatments. There was no significant relationship between changes in disease severity status and the amount of money spent monthly on alternative treatments (*P* = .196).

Household Income

There was a significant relationship between disease severity and household income (*P*<.0001). Patients with higher disease severity levels had lower household incomes. After conducting the regression analysis for both the combination of insurance with out-of-pocket expenditures and out-of-pocket expenditures alone, no significant association was noted between household income and the total amount (out of pocket plus insurance) of money spent (*P* = .258) or household income and out-of-pocket money spent (*P* = .462).

Gender

Patients were grouped by gender to evaluate differences in expenditures between men and women. No significant differences were noted between the genders for out-of-pocket expenditures (*P* = .553) and total expenditures including insurance (*P* = .472).

DISCUSSION

Total treatment cost (including insurance and out-of-pocket expenses) per month increased with

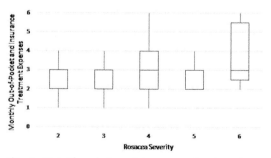

Fig. 2. Out-of-pocket and insurance treatment expenses. Monthly out of pocket and insurance treatment expenses based on rosacea severity category. Expenses: 1, no expenses; 2, less than $25; 3, $25 to $50; 4, $51 to $100; 5, $101 to $200; 6, more than $200.

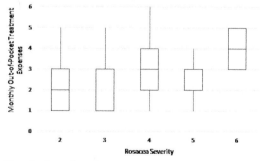

Fig. 3. Out-of-pocket treatment expenses. Monthly out-of-pocket treatment expenses based on rosacea severity category. Expenses: 1, no expenses; 2, less than $10; 3, $10 to $25; 4, $26 to $50; 5, $51 to $100; 6, greater than $100.

increasing disease severity, suggesting that patients are motivated to control their disease. This finding parallels that of a treatment cost survey study pertaining to psoriasis patients. There was a significant relationship between total and out-of-pocket expenses to manage psoriasis and severity of disease. The expense of managing psoriasis is higher in patients with more severe disease.[1] In this study, severe disease was associated with lower household incomes. This finding suggests that patients with lower household incomes are spending more money out of pocket and have higher insurance expenditures for rosacea treatment. The authors' study did not examine specific insurance plans or coverage options; however, future studies could examine individual benefits and evaluate rosacea severity among individuals with similar insurance plans. Such studies could inform the need for better coverage options, especially if increased severity predominates among lower income households.

Ensuring that patients are receiving the most efficacious treatments is crucial. Although there are a plethora of rosacea treatment options, only a few have strong data demonstrating efficacy.[2] This study offers a snapshot of expenditures and severity; it does not provide insight into changes in severity with continued use of medications or other therapies. Familiarization of evidence-based clinical recommendations and consensus guidelines may equip physicians to educate patients about the most efficacious and cost-effective treatment options to assist patients in making cost-conscious decisions in the management of their rosacea.[3]

DISCLOSURE STATEMENT

S.R. Feldman is a speaker for Janssen and Taro. He is a consultant and speaker for Galderma, Stiefel/GlaxoSmithKline, Abbott Labs, Leo Pharma Inc. S.R. Feldman has received grants from Galderma, Janssen, Abbott Labs, Amgen, Stiefel/GlaxoSmithKline, Celgene and Anacor. He is a consultant for Amgen, Baxter, Caremark, Gerson Lehrman Group, Guidepoint Global, Hanall Pharmaceutical Co Ltd, Kikaku, Lilly, Merck & Co Inc, Merz Pharmaceuticals, Mylan, Novartis Pharmaceuticals, Pfizer Inc, Qurient, Suncare Research, and Xenoport. He is on an advisory board for Pfizer Inc. S.R. Feldman is the founder and holds stock in Causa Research and holds stock and is majority owner in Medical Quality Enhancement Corporation. He receives Royalties from UpToDate and Xlibris. J.G. Turbeville, H. Alinia, S.M. Tuchayi, N. Bahrami, L.A. Cardwell, O. Awosika, I. Richardson, and K.E. Huang have no conflicts to disclose.

REFERENCES

1. Feldman SR, Fleischer AB, Reboussin DM, et al. The economic impact of psoriasis increases with psoriasis severity. J Am Acad Dermatol 1997;37:564–9. Available at: http://www.ncbi.nlm.nih.gov/pubmed/9344194. Accessed September 5, 2016.

2. van Zuuren EJ, Kramer S, Carter B, et al. Interventions for rosacea. In: van Zuuren EJ, editor. Cochrane database syst rev. Chichester (United Kingdom): John Wiley & Sons, Ltd; 2011. p. CD003262. Available at: http://www.ncbi.nlm.nih.gov/pubmed/21412882. Accessed August 26, 2017.

3. Schaller M, Almeida LMC, Bewley A, et al. Rosacea treatment update: recommendations from the global ROSacea COnsensus (ROSCO) panel. Br J Dermatol 2017;176:465–71. Available at: http://www.ncbi.nlm.nih.gov/pubmed/27861741. Accessed August 26, 2017.

Coping Mechanisms and Resources for Patients Suffering from Rosacea

Leah A. Cardwell, MD[a],*, Timothy Nyckowski, BS[a],
Laura N. Uwakwe, MD[a], Steven R. Feldman, MD, PhD[a,b,c]

KEYWORDS

- Psychosocial • Quality of life • Support • Disease burden

KEY POINTS

- Rosacea is a dermatologic condition with significant quality-of-life and psychosocial impact.
- Patients may seek psychosocial support and coping mechanisms for rosacea, and physicians can help empower patients by being aware of available resources.
- Coping mechanisms and resources may optimize quality-of-life and psychosocial impact outcomes in patients with rosacea.

INTRODUCTION

The face has major significance in nearly every facet of human interaction, including social relationships, romantic life, and business relationships. Rosacea is a chronic, relapsing dermatologic condition that has a profound impact on how patients view themselves, how others view patients, and how patients believe others view them. Rosacea sufferers may experience social stigmatization and psychosocial detriment.[1] Rosacea is a highly impactful condition is associated with depression, anxiety, embarrassment, social phobia, and stress.[1–7] the authors highlight the resources available to rosacea patients.

METHODS

MEDLINE and PsycINFO databases were searched to identify articles pertaining to rosacea coping resources. The term "rosacea" was searched in combination with "patient resources," "coping," "dealing with," "blog," "forum," "support," "nonpharmacologic," and "psychological." The authors assumed the patients' perspective by searching all available links pertaining to rosacea coping resources within the first 10 pages of a Google query with the aforementioned terms. Results that were linked to organizations with clear financial incentives to providing patient resources were excluded.

RESULTS

Biopsychosocial Approach to Rosacea Management

In approaching patients with chronic dermatologic conditions, several resources advocated a biopsychosocial approach, understanding that rosacea may affect social status, romantic relationships, and self-esteem.[8–12] A biopsychosocial approach considers that there may be a wide

---

Disclosure: See last page of article.
[a] Department of Dermatology, Center for Dermatology Research, Wake Forest School of Medicine, Medical Center Boulevard, Winston-Salem, NC 27157-1071, USA; [b] Department of Pathology, Wake Forest School of Medicine, Medical Center Boulevard, Winston-Salem, NC 27157-1071, USA; [c] Department of Social Sciences & Health Policy, Wake Forest School of Medicine, Medical Center Boulevard, Winston-Salem, NC 27157-1071, USA
* Corresponding author.
E-mail address: lcardwell06@gmail.com

Dermatol Clin 36 (2018) 171–174
https://doi.org/10.1016/j.det.2017.11.013
0733-8635/18/© 2017 Elsevier Inc. All rights reserved.

range of psychological sequelae among rosacea patients. This approach establishes a therapeutic atmosphere that is both empathetic and reassuring. Practitioners inquire about quality-of-life impact and validate patients' distress.[12] Physician acknowledgment that patients' psychosocial status may be negatively impacted by rosacea could motivate patients to openly discuss their experiences.[13] Differences between a patient's assessment of disease severity and a provider's assessment of disease severity may suggest that a patient is experiencing psychosocial detriment due to their rosacea.[13] Patients may experience a substantial improvement in quality of life by acknowledging the chronic, relapsing nature of the condition.[14]

Patient Educational Resources

Multiple websites provide patients with information about the cause, pathogenesis, symptoms, clinical features, triggers, and treatment options for rosacea.[15–20] This information is presented as patient-friendly material without extensive medical jargon. A rosacea diary, available through the National Rosacea Society, allows patients to log their rosacea flares and identify triggers.[21] This resource may be a source of empowerment for patients because they are able to use their entries in collaboration with their dermatologist and as a means to limit rosacea flares.

Online Social Support Communities

People with chronic disease who do not have strong personal support networks are especially likely to use online social support systems to fulfill social needs.[22] Online sources allow for increased information sharing of disease-specific knowledge and can empower patients.[22] For individuals that prefer anonymity, there are specialized online forums that discuss the emotional nuances of rosacea and ways to cope.[23,24] Online support groups may be the most widely used social platform in chronic disease management, offering patients peer support, social acceptance, understanding, and validation.[22] Since patients may not feel comfortable discussing certain topics with their physician, these social media outlets may serve as a more comfortable forum to share experiences and concerns.[25] Contemporary social site use in patients with chronic disease can improve patient care by providing social, emotional, or experiential support.[26,27] Social media platforms, such as Facebook, have dedicated rosacea support groups, providing a sense of community.[28–30] These social network sites have more active users than standard online support groups (**Table 1**).[22]

DISCUSSION

Since dermatologic conditions may be directly visible to the public, they tend to have significant psychosocial and quality of life impact. An international study on implicit association that included 6831 participants from 8 countries confirmed that the facial erythema of rosacea is strongly associated with perception of poor health and negative personality traits.[31] Individuals with erythematous rosacea are less likely to be perceived, on initial impression, as relaxed, healthy, and well.[31] Patients that have more severe physical symptoms tend to have more severe psychological symptoms.[2–5] In a retrospective study assessing 608 million dermatology visits, the odds ratio for depressive disease in patients with rosacea was 4.81.[2] Anxiety, embarrassment, social phobia, and stress are common comorbidities in rosacea sufferers.[1,4–6]

Patient education improves quality of life of those living with chronic inflammatory skin conditions.[32,33] Physicians might consider routinely providing rosacea patients with educational materials to clarify and emphasize the importance of treatment adherence and establish realistic treatment goals.[34] By fully understanding the chronic, relapsing nature of rosacea, patients may be better equipped to cope with the frustration of symptom recurrence. Enhancing self-efficacy, a person's perceived capability to perform actions required to achieve concrete goals, leads to improved motivation, behaviors, patterns of thought, and emotional well-being.[35] Self-efficacy, a significant determinant of coping ability, can be enhanced by critically analyzing the cause of physiologic symptoms and persuading the patient to adhere to behavioral changes, such as trigger avoidance and treatment compliance, which may modify the course of rosacea.[35,36] By providing rosacea patients with educational and social support, patient self-efficacy may be enhanced. Self-efficacy has been instrumental in optimizing coping ability in several chronic ailments, including chronic pain, fibromyalgia, and irritable bowel disease.[37–39] Patients may not feel comfortable fully disclosing their concerns to their physician. In these instances, an online community setting or forum may be beneficial.[26]

Patients with limited access to or knowledge of the Internet may have trouble using the resources mentioned in this review. Even with ideal medical therapy, rosacea is a chronic disease that often relapses. Although this condition is not medically dire, it may cause considerable psychosocial distress.[40] Physicians who are aware of coping resources for patients may be better equipped to optimize patients' outcomes.

Table 1
Resources for rosacea patients

Online literature	National Rosacea Society https://www.rosacea.org/patients/materials/understanding/index.php International Rosacea Foundation http://www.internationalrosaceafoundation.org/ American Academy of Dermatology https://www.aad.org/public/diseases/acne-and-rosacea/rosacea American Osteopathic College of Dermatology http://www.aocd.org/?page=Rosacea British Skin Foundation http://www.britishskinfoundation.org.uk/SkinInformation/AtoZofSkindisease/ Rosacea.aspx American Academy of Family Physicians http://www.aafp.org/afp/2015/0801/p187.html

Social media
  network-based
  forums
	Facebook—Rosacea Awareness
	https://www.facebook.com/RosaceaAwareness
	Facebook—National Rosacea Society
	https://www.facebook.com/nationalrosaceasociety/
	Facebook—Rosacea Support Group
	https://www.facebook.com/rosaceasupportgroup/

Online forms	Rosacea Support Group https://rosacea-support.org/ Experience My Rosacea http://experiencemyrosacea.co.uk/ Reddit—Rosacea https://www.reddit.com/r/Rosacea/

DISCLOSURE STATEMENT

S.R. Feldman is a speaker for Janssen and Taro. He is a consultant and speaker for Galderma, Stiefel/GlaxoSmithKline, Abbott Labs, Leo Pharma Inc. S.R. Feldman has received grants from Galderma, Janssen, Abbott Labs, Amgen, Stiefel, GlaxoSmithKline, Celgene, and Anacor. He is a consultant for Amgen, Baxter, Caremark, Gerson Lehrman Group, Guidepoint Global, Hanall Pharmaceutical Co Ltd, Kikaku, Lilly, Merck & Co Inc, Merz Pharmaceuticals, Mylan, Novartis Pharmaceuticals, Pfizer Inc, Qurient, Suncare Research, and Xenoport. He is on an advisory board for Pfizer Inc. S.R. Feldman is the founder and holds stock in Causa Research and holds stock and is majority owner in Medical Quality Enhancement Corporation. He receives royalties from UpToDate and Xlibris. L.A. Cardwell, T. Nyckowski, and L.N. Uwakwe have nothing to disclose.

REFERENCES

1. Moustafa F, Lewallen RS, Feldman SR. The psychological impact of rosacea and the influence of current management options. J Am Acad Dermatol 2014;71:973–80.

2. Gupta MA, Gupta AK, Chen SJ, et al. Comorbidity of rosacea and depression: an analysis of the National Ambulatory Medical Care Survey and National Hospital Ambulatory Care Survey–Outpatient Department data collected by the U.S. National Center for Health Statistics from 1995 to 2002. Br J Dermatol 2005;153:1176–81.

3. Bohm D, Schwanitz P, Stock Gissendanner S, et al. Symptom severity and psychological sequelae in rosacea: results of a survey. Psychol Health Med 2014; 19:586–91.

4. Egeberg A, Hansen PR, Gislason GH, et al. Patients with rosacea have increased risk of depression and anxiety disorders: a Danish Nationwide Cohort Study. Dermatology 2016;232:208–13.

5. Orzechowska A, Talarowska M, Zboralski K, et al. Subjective evaluation of symptoms and effects of treatment and the intensity of the stress and anxiety levels among patients with selected diseases of the skin and gastrointestinal tract. Psychiatr Pol 2013; 47:225–37 [in Polish].

6. Drummond PD, Su D. Blushing in rosacea sufferers. J Psychosom Res 2012;72:153–8.

7. Tan J, Berg M. Rosacea: current state of epidemiology. J Am Acad Dermatol 2013;69:S27–35.

8. Orion E, Wolf R. Psychologic factors in the development of facial dermatoses. Clin Dermatol 2014;32:763–6.

9. Fried RG. Nonpharmacologic treatments in psychodermatology. Dermatol Clin 2002;20:177–85.

10. Wolf JEJ. Medication adherence: a key factor in effective management of rosacea. Adv Ther 2001; 18:272–81.

11. Fava GA, Cosci F, Sonino N. Current psychosomatic practice. Psychother Psychosom 2017;86: 13–30.

12. Ghosh S, Behere RV, Sharma P, et al. Psychiatric evaluation in dermatology: an overview. Indian J Dermatol 2013;58:39–43.

13. Gupta MA, Gupta AK. Psychiatric and psychological co-morbidity in patients with dermatologic disorders: epidemiology and management. Am J Clin Dermatol 2003;4:833–42.

14. Tuckman A. The potential psychological impact of skin conditions. Dermatol Ther (Heidelb) 2017;7: 53–7.

15. Rosacea | American Academy of Dermatology. Available at: https://www.aad.org/public/diseases/acne-and-rosacea/rosacea. Accessed September 6, 2017.

16. Rosacea. Available at: http://www.britishskinfoundation.org.uk/SkinInformation/AtoZofSkindisease/Rosacea.aspx. Accessed September 6, 2017.

17. American Academy of Family Physicians. LK, Herbert L. Muncie J, Phillips-Savoy AR. American family physician. Am Fam Physician American Academy of Family Physicians; 1970. Available at: http://www.aafp.org/afp/2015/0801/p187.html Accessed September 6, 2017.

18. Understanding Rosacea | Rosacea.org. Available from: https://www.rosacea.org/patients/materials/understanding/index.php Accessed September 6, 2017.

19. Rosacea - American Osteopathic College of Dermatology (AOCD). Available from: http://www.aocd.org/?page=Rosacea. Accessed September 6, 2017.

20. Rosacea Treatments - International Rosacea Foundation. Available from: http://www.internationalrosaceafoundation.org/. Accessed September 6, 2017.

21. Rosacea Diary Booklet | Rosacea.org. Available from: https://www.rosacea.org/patients/materials/diary/index.php. Accessed September 6, 2017.

22. Merolli M, Gray K, Martin-Sanchez F. Health outcomes and related effects of using social media in chronic disease management: a literature review and analysis of affordances. J Biomed Inform 2013;46:957–69. Available at: http://www.ncbi.nlm.nih.gov/pubmed/23702104. Accessed August 29, 2017.

23. Rosacea Support Group. Where the rosacea community meets online: rosacea support group. Available at: https://rosacea-support.org/. Accessed September 6, 2017.

24. Experience My Rosacea. Available from: http://experiencemyrosacea.co.uk/. Accessed September 6, 2017.

25. Alinia H, Moradi Tuchayi S, Farhangian ME, et al. Rosacea patients seeking advice: qualitative analysis of patients' posts on a rosacea support forum. J Dermatolog Treat 2016;27:99–102.

26. Patel R, Chang T, Greysen SR, et al. Social media use in chronic disease: a systematic review and novel taxonomy. Am J Med 2015;128:1335–50.

27. Rosacea. Available at: https://www.reddit.com/r/Rosacea/. Accessed September 6, 2017.

28. Rosacea Support Group. Available at: https://www.facebook.com/rosaceasupportgroup/. Accessed September 6, 2017.

29. National Rosacea Society. Available at: https://www.facebook.com/nationalrosaceasociety/. Accessed June 28, 2017.

30. Rosacea Awareness. Available from: https://www.facebook.com/RosaceaAwareness/. Accessed June 28, 2017.

31. Dirschka T, Micali G, Papadopoulos L, et al. Perceptions on the psychological impact of facial erythema associated with rosacea: results of international survey. Dermatol Ther (Heidelb) 2015;5: 117–27.

32. Anderson R, Barbara A, Feldman S. What patients want: a content analysis of key qualities that influence patient satisfaction. J Med Pract Manage 2007;22:255–61.

33. de Bes J, Legierse CM, Prinsen CAC, et al. Patient education in chronic skin diseases: a systematic review. Acta Derm Venereol 2011;91:12–7.

34. Feldman SR, Sandoval L. Practice gap in patient education: comment on "the person-centered dermatology self-care index". Arch Dermatol 2012;148: 1255–6.

35. Ritter PL, Lorig K. The English and Spanish Self-Efficacy to Manage Chronic Disease Scale measures were validated using multiple studies. J Clin Epidemiol 2014;67:1265–73.

36. Jensen MP, Turner JA, Romano JM. Self-efficacy and outcome expectancies: relationship to chronic pain coping strategies and adjustment. Pain 1991; 44:263–9.

37. Jackson T, Wang Y, Wang Y, et al. Self-efficacy and chronic pain outcomes: a meta-analytic review. J Pain 2014;15:800–14.

38. Van Liew C, Brown KC, Cronan TA, et al. Predictors of pain and functioning over time in fibromyalgia syndrome: an autoregressive path analysis. Arthritis Care Res (Hoboken) 2013;65:251–6.

39. Keefer L, Kiebles JL, Taft TH. The role of self-efficacy in inflammatory bowel disease management: preliminary validation of a disease-specific measure. Inflamm Bowel Dis 2011;17:614–20.

40. Wehausen B, Hill DE, Feldman SR. Most people with psoriasis or rosacea are not being treated: a large population study. Dermatol Online J 2016;22 [pii: 13030/qt4nc3p4q2].

Moving?

Make sure your subscription moves with you!

To notify us of your new address, find your **Clinics Account Number** (located on your mailing label above your name), and contact customer service at:

Email: journalscustomerservice-usa@elsevier.com

800-654-2452 (subscribers in the U.S. & Canada)
314-447-8871 (subscribers outside of the U.S. & Canada)

Fax number: 314-447-8029

Elsevier Health Sciences Division
Subscription Customer Service
3251 Riverport Lane
Maryland Heights, MO 63043

*To ensure uninterrupted delivery of your subscription, please notify us at least 4 weeks in advance of move.

ELSEVIER

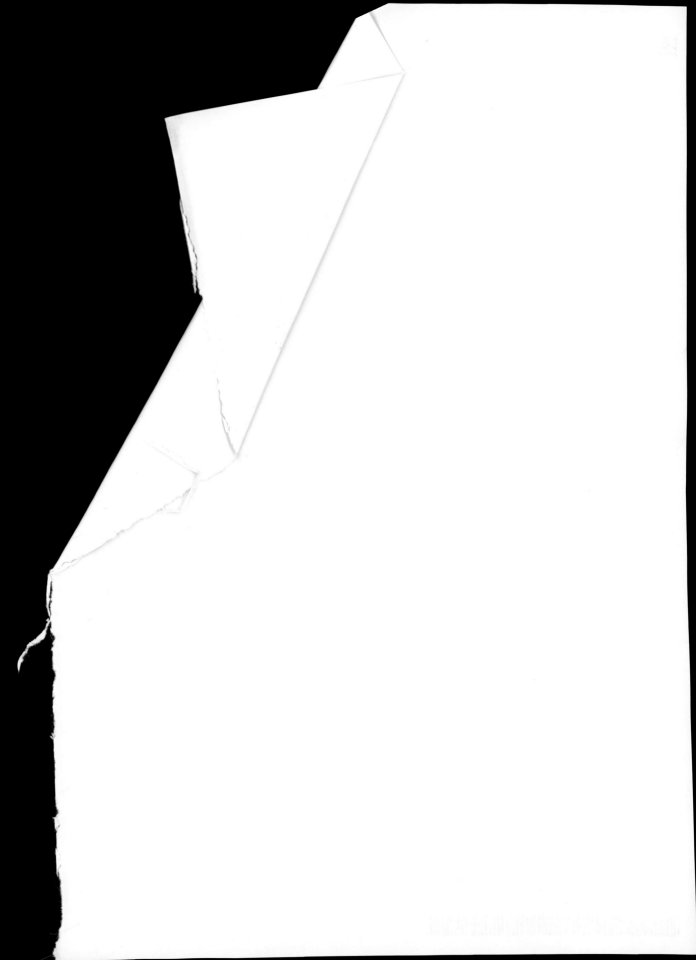

Printed and bound by CPI Group (UK) Ltd, Croydon, CR0 4YY

03/10/2024

01040383-0018

Printed and bound by CPI Group (UK) Ltd, Croydon, CR0 4YY

03/10/2024

01040383-0018